PHARMACOLOGY - RESEARCH, SAFETY TESTING AND REGULATION

OPIOIDS

PHARMACOLOGY, CLINICAL USES AND ADVERSE EFFECTS

PHARMACOLOGY - RESEARCH, SAFETY TESTING AND REGULATION

Additional books in this series can be found on Nova's website
under the Series tab.

Additional E-books in this series can be found on Nova's website
under the E-books tab.

PAIN MANAGEMENT – RESEARCH AND TECHNOLOGY

Additional books in this series can be found on Nova's website
under the Series tab.

Additional E-books in this series can be found on Nova's website
under the E-books tab.

PHARMACOLOGY - RESEARCH, SAFETY TESTING AND REGULATION

OPIOIDS

PHARMACOLOGY, CLINICAL USES AND ADVERSE EFFECTS

DJAVAKHI TVILDIANI
AND
KAKHA GEGECHKORI
EDITORS

Nova Science Publishers, Inc.
New York

For permission to use material from this book please contact us:
Telephone 631-231-7269; Fax 631-231-8175
Web Site: http://www.novapublishers.com

Library of Congress Cataloging-in-Publication Data

ISBN 978-1-61942-101-1
Library of Congress Control Number: 2011946169

Published by Nova Science Publishers, Inc. † New York

CONTENTS

PREFACE

Opioids are among the oldest and most enduring substances used for the management of pain and other medical problems. It is now known that the properties of the naturally occurring opioids (primarily morphine and codeine) and the related endogenous opioid-like peptides and synthetic chemical substances can be attributed to action at the receptors to which they bind within the central and peripheral nervous systems. This book presents current research in the study of the pharmacology, clinical uses and adverse effects of opioids. Topics include an historic review of the pain concepts and treatment by opioids; u-opioid receptor modulation of oxytocin and vasopressin release in the hypothalmic-neurohupophysial system and synergy abilities of spinal opioid receptors.

Chapter 1 - Sleep disordered breathing (SDB) associated with chronic opioid use is a diagnostic and therapeutic challenge for the clinician. Chronic opioid use is associated with sleep disturbances, excessive daytime sleepiness and daytime fatigue. Studies have shown that chronic opioid use is associated with respiratory complications including breathing instability during sleep, obstructive sleep apnea (OSA) central sleep apnea (CSA), or death.

The use of opioids has increased dramatically in recent years due to ~~an~~ increased awareness in the treatment of chronic pain amongst health professionals as well as patients. Pain control is essential in those who are suffering. However, it is important to recognize the effects of chronic opioids on sleep architecture as well as respiratory-related complications during sleep. Guidelines are lacking on how to recognize individuals at risk for respiratory complications during sleep, and how to effectively treat sleep disordered breathing in individuals who are affected.

Chapter 2 - Even though we already know from physiological studies that special receptors are responsible for conducting pain sensations to the brain, the phenomenon of pain still remains a medical and social problem. For centuries, physicians were helpless in the battle against pain. They could ease pain sensations with a few drugs, but they could not eliminate it. However, humankind struggled against pain from the very beginning, for thousands of years. As time went on, he used of medicinal herbs in the form of soporific sponges, opium juices and extracts from henbane. Particularly, at the close of the Middle Ages doctors had learnt to put their patients to sleep with pan relieving extracts obtained from the root and fruits mandrake, one of the oldest medicinal plants known to man, also known as mandragora. But until the 19th century pharmacy did not have some sort of effective drugs for pain relief. As early as 1806, the German pharmacist F.W. Sertürner succeeded in deriving an alkaloid from opium for the fight against pain, which he called "morphine", after the Greek god Morpheus. This was a reversion to the antique origins of medicine, in existence at the time of Hippocrates and his medical school, the juice of the poppy, opium were used for relieve pain, fever and insomnia. Knowledge of this drug, which in Greece and the Middles East was easy to obtain from the poppy, remained in use in popular medicine for centuries. This article provides historical perspective on pain concepts and evolution of pain therapy.

Chapter 3 - The Hypothalamic-Neurohypophysial System (HNS) in mammals controls diuresis and parturition through the release of the neuropeptides arginine-vasopressin (AVP) and oxytocin (OT). These neuropeptides are synthesized in hypothalamic Magnocellular neurons (MCNs) and are secreted into the blood stream from terminals in the neuro-hypophysis (NH). Neuroendocrine function in the HNS is modulated by opioids, either released endogenously or applied exogenously, by acting on μ- or κ-selective opioid receptors. Parturition is disrupted and the milk ejection reflex is inhibited during lactation when OT release is interrupted by opiate drugs. Also, water and salt balance are regulated by centrally or peripherally administered opioids acting on the HNS.

Mu- and kappa- opioid receptors have been identified in the soma and nerve endings of MCN using pharmacological and autoradiographic techniques. When activated in NH terminals, opioid receptors differentially inhibit various types of voltage-gated calcium channels (VGCC), hence modulating the amount of OT and/or AVP being released. In the present research, we characterized the expression of both μ- or κ-opioid receptors and VGCCs using immunocytochemical techniques and provide evidence for a differential targeting of channels in OT *vs.* AVP nerve terminals. We propose a model that can explain how opiate effects on VGCCs can directly mediate differences in the control of neurohypophysial OT and/or AVP release.

Chapter 4 - Reduced clinical efficacy of opioid analgesic drugs in chronic pain, including neuropathic pain, remains an unsolved issue. Since the spinal dorsal horn is a major site of opioid pain modulation, new insights into molecular opioid mechanisms may provide novel avenues for chronic therapy.

The reported experimental evidence supports the view that the efficacy of opioid ligands to depress nociceptive neurotransmission in dorsal horn neurons may be modified as a result of interaction with other receptors in the same family as well as with other receptor families. In this chapter we review conditions for potential interactions in a variety of experimental models.

Available data from two experimental models of pathological pain, namely the long-term potentiation of spinal C fiber-evoked potentials and surgical ligature of the fifth spinal nerve, support that spinal hyperexcitation may activate an endogenous factor that can enhance the effectiveness of spinally acting opioid ligands. Further, the spinal mu or delta opioid receptors undergo profound functional changes as a result of peripheral nerve injury, which are largely yet not exclusively attributable to tonic co-activation of the mu opioid receptor. Potentially involved mechanisms based on receptor-interactions as well as possible implications are discussed.

Chapter 5 - This chapter presents a concise overview of the pharmacology, clinical uses, and adverse effects of morphine-like drugs ('opioids'). Morphine, a natural product whose beneficial therapeutic use was discovered serendipitously thousands of years ago, remains the 'gold standard' for the relief of moderate to severe pain. Following the elucidation of morphine's chemical structure at the beginning of the 19th century and subsequent extensive design, synthesis, and testing of chemical analogs by pharmaceutical and academic laboratories, today there are multiple opioids available to the clinician. Although each is morphine-like and shares certain fundamental characteristics with morphine, they each have particular features, the nuances of which influence their clinical use and usefulness.

Chapter 6 - Strong opioids are widely used for several types of pain, such as acute or chronic, and moderate to severe pain. However, there have been many reports which describe its side effects, such as nausea, vomiting, constipation, analgesia, addiction, etc. Therefore, efforts to overcome these side effects and increase their effectiveness are made. Specific mechanisms of several opioids which are newly developed are described here and future aspects of strategy for developing strong opioids are explained.

For example, hydromorphone has a strong analgesic effect, but because of its short acting duration and fluctuation of blood concentration, there is a possibility of addiction. Also, it is inappropriate for basal pain. Prolonged releasing hydromorphone is developed by osmotic-controlled release technology (Jurnista®), and this can be used basal pain as well as breakthrough pain. In addition, delayed gastrointestinal(GI) mobility with the use of opiods has been well known. Naloxone, which was added to oxycodone, acts as an antagonist of receptors in the GI system and can improve constipation symptoms, developed under the name of Targin®. Furthermore, new opioids are being developed to have synergistic analgesic action between the receptor and other pain related receptors such as a-adrenergic (Tapentadol®). Through these newly developing opioids, we can consider future aspects of opiods as well as concepts for medical pain therapy.

Chapter 7 - Analyses of opioid.-related molecules using genetically modified animals have clarified the mechanisms of the analgesic action of morphine, its related side-effects, and individual variabilities in sensitivity. In the present study, we examined the relationship between the dosage of analgesics, including opioids, required after major abdominal surgery and polymorphisms of an opioid metabolism-related gene, ATP-binding cassette, sub-family B (MDR/TAP), member 1 (*ABCB1*). We studied 129 patients (74 males, 55 females; aged 28-80 years old) who were administered analgesics, including opioids, for pain relief following major abdominal surgery and who provided informed consent. The analyses were performed using multivariate analysis, with $p < 0.05$ considered statistically significant. We found a significant association between analgesic requirements and *ABCB1* polymorphisms. Studies on gene polymorphisms associated with analgesic requirements are important for developing appropriate personalized treatments with less side-effects.

Chapter 8 - Polydrug use is common among patients in opioid maintenance programs. Heroin users often abuse alcohol, which may deteriorate the outcome of opioid maintenance treatment.

Excessive alcohol consumption among opioid maintenance patients has been associated with quality of life impairments and with serious social and health costs. Patients who are dependent both on illicit drugs and alcohol may have a poorer treatment outcome than patients without alcohol problems. The clinical and psychosocial treatment of these patients presents challenging work for the clinician. Therefore, treatment outcomes may be further improved if clinical subtypes of substance abusers could be identified and matched to an adequate treatment program.

In this study we aim to assess the prevalence of a drinking problem and analyze the cognitive and behavioral features of problematic alcohol use in opioid addicts according to Cloninger and Lesch's alcoholism typologies in a sample of 102 heroin-dependent patients in

Opioid Maintenance Treatment. This sample was selected in the Addiction Unit of the Psychiatric Service of Santa Maria University Hospital, in Lisbon-Portugal.

Results show that alcohol use and alcohol-related problems are frequent among heroin-dependent patients. Study clinical descriptors discriminate Cloninger's type I and type II drinking problem and confirm this binary alcoholism classification in this population. Heroin-dependent patients classified as Cloninger´s type II problem drinkers showed a more severe cognitive-behavior profile than those with a type I alcohol problem, concerning alcohol-taking situation prototypes, beliefs and expectancies about alcohol effects. Data only allows preliminary results about the Lesch's alcoholism classification

This cognitive and behavioral multidimensional assessment has relevant indicators to diagnose different drinking problems among the opioid maintenance programs population. It may improve intervention and treatment outcomes, reducing current health and psychosocial damage associated with an alcohol-abusing lifestyle.

In: Opioids: Pharmacology, Clinical Uses and Adverse Effects ISBN 978-1-61942-101-1
Editors: Djavakhi Tvildiani and Kakha Gegechkori

Chapter 1

CHRONIC OPIOID USE: EFFECTS ON RESPIRATION AND SLEEP

Michelle Cao[1] and Shahrokh Javaheri[2,3]
[1]Stanford Sleep Disorders Clinic, Stanford University, Redwood City, California, US
[2]Division of Pulmonary, Critical Care, Sleep Medicine, University of Cincinnati College of Medicine, Mason, Ohio, US
[3]Medical Director, Sleepcare Diagnostics, Mason, Ohio, US

ABSTRACT

Sleep disordered breathing (SDB) associated with chronic opioid use is a diagnostic and therapeutic challenge for the clinician. Chronic opioid use is associated with sleep disturbances, excessive daytime sleepiness and daytime fatigue. Studies have shown that chronic opioid use is associated with respiratory complications including breathing instability during sleep, obstructive sleep apnea (OSA) central sleep apnea (CSA), or death.

The use of opioids has increased dramatically in recent years due to ~~an~~ increased awareness in the treatment of chronic pain amongst health professionals as well as patients. Pain control is essential in those who are suffering. However, it is important to recognize the effects of chronic opioids on sleep architecture as well as respiratory-related complications during sleep. Guidelines are lacking on how to recognize individuals at risk for respiratory complications during sleep, and how to effectively treat sleep disordered breathing in individuals who are affected.

INTRODUCTION

Pain is a national and public health challenge. Recent data from the Institute of Medicine (IOM) reports that chronic pain affects at least 116 million adults in the United States. [1] A joint USA Today, ABC News, and Stanford University Medical Center poll in 2005 indicated that 19% of American adults, or 1 out of 5, suffer from chronic pain. There is growing recognition of chronic pain syndrome and a movement towards aggressively treating this condition. A joint statement by the American Pain Society and the American Academy of Pain Medicine in 1997 emphasized and supported the use of opioids for the treatment of chronic pain, with minimal associated respiratory risks.

For years, opioids have been a significant component in the treatment of chronic pain. In recent years however, opioid use has increased dramatically due to an increased awareness by health care providers to treat chronic pain more effectively and patients are encouraged to seek treatment. The recognition for more aggressive treatment of chronic pain has contributed to a rise in extended use of opioids. Moreover, aside from its use for pain, opioids are commonly used in the treatment of Restless Legs Syndrome as well as in the post-operative surgical setting.

The increased prevalence of chronic opioid use has made sleep related breathing disorders secondary to opioids a significant health related issue. Chronic opioid use is associated with sleep disturbances, daytime hypersomnolence and daytime fatigue. Studies have shown that chronic opioid use is associated with respiratory complications including instability of breathing during sleep, obstructive sleep apnea (OSA), and central sleep apnea (CSA). Several studies have suggested the association between sudden death in patients on chronic opioid therapy. It is important to recognize effects of chronic opioids on sleep architecture, respiratory complications during sleep, and how to effectively treat sleep disordered breathing in individuals who are affected.

Prevalence of Opioid Use

From 1990 to 1996, the use of opioids has increased for four opioid analgesics; fentanyl, morphine, oxycodone, hydromorphone by 1168%, 59%, 23%, and 19%, respectively. [2] Methadone maintenance treatment programs (MMT) are also on the rise. From 1997 to 2003, therapeutic use of methadone and oxycodone has increased by 824 and 660%, respectively. [3] From 1992 to 2008, substance abuse treatment admissions for those age 50 or older rose from 6.6% to 12.2%. [4]

In addition, an estimated 4.7 million individuals are using opioids illegally. A 2005 study showed that 9.5% of 12th graders used Vicodin, and 5.5% of these students used OxyContin. [5] Prescription painkillers significantly contribute to the total number of drug related deaths. In 2007, about 28,000 Americans died from unintentional drug poisoning, and of these, 12,000 died from prescription painkillers. [6]

Moreover, opioids are routinely used in surgical patients in the post-operative setting. This contributes to increased post-operative risk of respiratory complications in predisposed individuals, such as those with preexisting OSA. Overall, the increased used of opioids has resulted in increased morbidity and mortality. [7]

Opioid Receptors

Opioid receptors are a family of G-protein coupled receptors (GPCRs). Ligand binding of opioid receptors activates inhibitory intracellular pathways leading to a reduction in neuronal excitability. There are four classes of opioid receptors; δ (DOP) receptor, μ (MOP) receptor, κ

(KOP) receptor, and nociceptin/orphanin FQ peptide (NOP) receptor. Each receptor is associated with one or more endogenous ligands including endorphins, enkephalins, dynorphins, and nociceptin/orphanin. The endogenous opioid system participates in mediating physiologic responses such as pain, respiratory control, stress, appetite, and thermoregulation.

Opioid receptors are found in both central and peripheral nervous systems. They are abundant in respiratory control centers including the brainstem, insula, thalamus, and anterior cingulate cortex. Peripherally, they are located in carotid bodies. Endogenous and μ (MOP) opioid receptors are found in the respiratory centers in the pons and medulla. [8] Most of the clinically used opioids are selective for the μ receptor. Stimulation of μ and κ receptors in particular, is associated with respiratory depression. [9]

Respiratory Rhythm Generation

Experimental studies in neonatal rats have improved our understanding of how respiration is controlled. Discovered in 1990, there are two distinct respiratory rhythm generators located in the ventrolateral medullary portion of the neonatal rat brainstem. [10] [11] These two distinct complexes are known as the pre-Botzinger complex (pre-BotC) and the retrotrapezoid nucleus/parafacial respiratory group (RTN/pFRC), which are normally coupled and generate normal respiratory rhythm. [12] The pre-BotC is responsible for inspiratory rhythm generation, while the RTN/pFRC is responsible for expiratory rhythm generation. The respiratory rhythm in these complexes persists en bloc and in slices after attenuation of postsynaptic inhibition, supporting the hypothesis that intrinsic rhythmic pacemaker neurons located in these complexes drive the respiratory rhythm. [11] These findings have not been replicated in humans.

Respiratory Rhythm Generation and μ-Opioid Receptor

Opioids affect the pre-BotC and RTN/pFRG preferentially. The pre-BotC is active during inspiration and is inhibited by opioids, whereas the RTN/pFRG is active during expiration and is insensitive to opioids. DAMGO, a μ opioid agonist, when applied to rat brainstem containing only the pre-BotC, resulted in a dose dependent lengthening of inspiratory periods, consequently slowing down the respiratory rate. [11] When the same μ opioid agonist was applied to rat brainstem containing both the pre-BotC and RTN/pFRG, respiratory rate slowed down but also became irregular due to skipped breaths. When the pre-BotC is depressed, respiratory rhythm generation is taken over by the RTN/pFRG. [12] [13]

Mellen and colleagues described a "quantal" respiratory pattern that is similar to the pattern seen in Mobitz type II second-degree heart block, in which there are regular skipped beats throughout the cardiac rhythm. [13] As described above, when DAMGO was applied to rat brainstem containing both the pre-BotC and RTN/pFRG, the respiratory rhythm slowed but also showed increased inspiratory periods due to skipped inspirations, and so the breathing rhythm became irregular. Although the skipped breaths represented intermittent attenuation of output from the pre-BotC, the authors found that sub threshold action potentials were still present. This was named "quantal" respiratory pattern because the action potentials remained regular but were not completely transmitted.

The pre-BotC appears to be the dominant sight for inspiration and contains neurokinin-1 receptor (NK1R) and μ opioid receptors. In neonatal rodents, stimulation with μ opioid agonists results in respiratory rate suppression. [14] Lesions in this area demonstrate apneas during sleep as well as an irregular breathing pattern during wakefulness and sleep. [11,15] [16] A study in adult rats showed that accumulative loss of pre-BotC NK1R neurons led to progressive disturbances in sleep related breathing initially in rapid eye movement (REM) sleep, followed by non-rapid eye movement (NREM) sleep, and with greater than 80% of neuronal loss, in wakefulness. The abnormal breathing events were characterized by central hypopneas and apneas, and when most severe, they were characterized as ataxic breathing. [16] [17]

An important study using adult rats identified that NK1R expressing pre-BotC neurons constitute the critical site in the medulla mediating opioid-induced respiratory rate suppression. [18] The anatomical region most strongly associated with slowing of respiratory rate corresponds to the pre-BotC as identified by NK1R expression and in vitro electrophysiology. In rhythmically active brainstem section in vitro, NK1R expressing pre-BotC neurons are selectively inhibited by opioids. Continuous local unilateral application of a μ opioid receptor agonist DAMGO or fentanyl into the pre-BotC caused sustained slowing of respiratory rate, increased respiratory rate variability (ataxic breathing), and suppressed genioglossus muscle activation. Interestingly, the reduction in respiratory rate was due to a prolonged expiratory time without change in inspiratory time. These changes were fully reversed by the μ opioid receptor antagonist naloxone. At sufficient concentrations of μ opioid agonists, complete cessation of breathing was seen as manifested by complete cessation of genioglossus and diaphragmatic muscle activity. By infusing a μ opioid agonist in conjunction with recording of muscle activity across sleep-wake states, the authors demonstrated that opioids cause a state-dependent respiratory rate depression that is most profound in deep non-REM sleep and during anesthesia. The authors speculate that the pre-BotC is fully responsible for respiratory rate suppression following systemic administration of opioid analgesics.

Opioids and Control of Respiration

The fundamental drive to breathe is located in the brainstem, which receives inputs from the cortex as well as central and peripheral chemoreceptors. Respiration is controlled by central respiratory pacemakers that are located in the brainstem and interact with central as well as peripheral chemoreceptors and mechanoreceptors. Chemosensory organs that monitor blood oxygen (PaO_2) and carbon dioxide ($PaCO_2$) concentrations are located in the brainstem (central chemoreceptors) and peripherally in carotid bodies (peripheral chemoreceptors). Central chemoreceptors (located in nucleus tractus solitaries, dorsal respiratory group, medullary raphe, pre-BotC, and RTN/pFRC) primarily sense the pH of the central nervous system (CNS), which directly correlates with resting carbon dioxide ($PaCO_2$) levels in the blood. [19] The degree of stimulation of the respiratory system for a given level of $PaCO_2$ and CNS pH is known as the hypercapnic ventilatory response (HCVR).

Peripheral chemoreceptors are located in the glomus cells of the carotid body, and are the main sensors of blood oxygen levels (PaO_2). [20] Peripheral chemoreceptors communicate with central respiratory generators, which have a direct effect on motor neurons that innervate respiratory muscles (i.e. diaphragm, intercostals, abdominal muscles). Carotid body chemoreceptors communicate with the nucleus tractus solitaries (NTS) located in the medulla, via the glossopharyngeal nerve and modulate respiration via direct connections between the NTS and the RTN/pFRG. The glomus cells of the carotid body are essential in mediating the hypoxic ventilatory response (HVR), the degree of respiratory stimulation for a given level of oxygen (PaO_2) in the blood. [9] Bilateral carotid body resection has been shown to abolish the HVR as well as HCVR in humans. [21] [22] [23]

Acute use of opioids can significantly decrease both the HCVR and HVR. In humans, acute morphine administration has been shown to depress the HVR. [24] [25] In healthy volunteers, by comparing HVR for intrathecal morphine versus intravenous morphine delivery, Bailey and colleagues demonstrated that acute morphine administration is likely to exert its depressant effect on the HVR by direct action on the brainstem rather than carotid bodies. [26] The authors theorize that opioids are likely to affect brainstem synapses between carotid body peripheral chemoreflexes with afferents to the NTS, which contains μ receptors. [27] [9] Acute ingestion of opioids has been shown to blunt the increase in respiratory drive associated with increased respiratory resistance. [28] Banzett and colleagues showed that acute administration of intravenous morphine profoundly reduced the sensation of dyspnea and the HCVR in normal healthy volunteers who are subjected to an environment that evoked a sense of air hunger. [29]

In contrast, with chronic opioid use subjects have shown reduced HCVR and an increased HVR. [28] In a study comparing 50 patients on chronic methadone (MMT) to 20 controls, the authors found that MMT patients had a blunted central (HCVR) and an elevated peripheral (HVR) chemoreceptor response. [30] It is hypothesized that this may be related to long-term stimulation of hypoxic response by long-term intermittent hypoxia. The authors also found that the respiratory rate rather than tidal volume change was the major physiologic response contributing to HCVR and HVR differences. A study by the same authors showed that concurrent chronic use of antidepressants and methadone may further reduce an already blunted HCVR leading to increased risk of central sleep apnea. [31] These patients had significantly reduced central chemosensitivity (HCVR) compared to patients taking methadone alone.

Opioids and Sleep

During sleep, the respiratory pattern in patients with chronic exposure to opioids is characterized as irregular with a mixture of central apneas, ataxic breathing (Biot's respiration), and frequent respiratory pauses. Camille Biot first described this irregular, ataxic breathing pattern in 1897 in a 16 year-old patient with tuberculous meningitis. [32] Biot's original illustration showed breathes of differing amplitude without any regular rhythm, but with random apneic periods of variable duration. Biot's breathing is associated with diseases of the central nervous system, damage to the medulla, high altitude pulmonary edema, as well as chronic opioid use. It is differentiated from Cheyne-Stokes respiration (a form of central sleep apnea seen in individuals with systolic heart failure or neurologic insult) by a lack of cyclical crescendo-decrescendo respiratory pattern. [33]

Aside from breathing disturbances during sleep, acute and chronic opioid exposure has been shown to adversely affect sleep architecture. Sleep is divided into two different stages; non-rapid eye movement sleep (NREM) and rapid eye movement sleep (REM). NREM sleep is further divided into 3 subsequent stages; N1, N2, and N3 (N3 is considered slow wave sleep). In humans, opioids affect sleep architecture by increasing the amount of NREM sleep while decreasing slow wave sleep and REM sleep.

In a case control study of 50 subjects on methadone maintenance treatment program (MMT), compared to controls, MMT subjects had significantly less stage REM and stage N1 sleep and more stage N2 sleep compared to normal subjects. [31] The study did not find differences in arousal index, total sleep time, or sleep efficiency between the comparison groups. [31] In another double-blind, placebo controlled crossover study on 42 healthy subjects, Dimsdale and colleagues showed that acute ingestion of sustained release morphine and methadone decreased stage N3 (slow wave sleep), increased stage N2, but had no effect on sleep efficiency, wake after sleep onset, and total sleep time. [34] A study from anesthesia perspective examined sleep architecture in 7 healthy, pain free subjects in response to intravenously administered morphine, and found that morphine led to reductions in stage N3 sleep and REM sleep, increased stage N2 sleep, but did not increase awakenings or arousals. [35] In a double-blind placebo controlled study, Bernards and colleagues examined respiratory pattern and sleep architecture in OSA patients by use of intravenous remifentanyl, a short-acting opioid that reaches steady state plasma concentrations in a timely manner. They found that remifentanyl increased stage N1, markedly decreased REM sleep, and decreased sleep efficiency. They also found an increased number of central apneas. [36]

Insomnia, sleep fragmentation, and a reduction in REM sleep have been shown in patients withdrawing from chronic opioids. This is followed by an increase in REM sleep, rebound stage N3, and increase in total sleep time. The rebound in stage N3 and REM sleep occurred between 13-22 weeks following chronic opioid withdrawal. [37-39] In an observational study by Howe and colleagues on acute heroin abstinence, there was an increase in wakefulness and a decrease in stage N3 and REM sleep. Total sleep time was decreased and continued to be below normal range even after 7 days of abstinence. [40-42]

Opioids and Breathing during Sleep

Sleep-disordered breathing (SDB) describes a specific group of sleep related disorders characterized by repeated interruptions of breathing during sleep resulting in hypoxemia, hypoventilation, autonomic activation, arousals, and disturbed sleep. Obstructive sleep apnea (OSA), a subset of SDB, is a highly prevalent condition characterized by repetitive episodes of upper airway collapse due to increased airflow resistance despite ongoing respiratory effort. In contrast, central sleep apnea (CSA) is characterized by disruption of central neurologic control on the drive to breathe leading to respiratory pauses. In contrast to obstructive sleep apnea, respiratory effort is abolished in central sleep apnea.

Breathing abnormalities during sleep associated with chronic opioid exposure was first reported in 2001. There are two physiologic conditions that contribute to the direct negative effect of opioids on the respiratory system during sleep; the loss of the wakefulness stimulus and skeletal muscle atonia associated with rapid eye movement (REM) sleep. Thresholds to arousal, hypercapnia, and hypoxemia are altered during REM sleep. The presence of opioids may further alter these thresholds, resulting in further increase partial pressure of carbon dioxide and decrease partial pressure of oxygen. In one study however, chronic opioid ingestion was associated with only mild decrease in arterial oxygen saturation and a mild increase in transcutaneous carbon dioxide tension. [31] Moreover, the activity of muscles of the upper airway and ~~of~~ accessory respiratory muscles are reduced during sleep but do not significantly alter airway resistance in normal individuals. However, in individuals with sleep disordered breathing opioids may further decrease the activity of these muscles, consequently increase airway resistance and worsening gas exchange.

Chronic opioid use is an established risk factor for the development of Studies have demonstrated that 30-90% of patients on chronic opioids have some form of sleep disordered breathing. A retrospective study of 98 individuals on chronic opioid medication for chronic pain found 36% had OSA, 24% had CSA, and 21% had combined OSA and CSA. [43] A larger cohort of 147 patients with chronic opioid use showed that 39% had OSA, 24% had CSA, and 8% had mixed OSA and CSA, similar to findings by Mogri et al. [44]

Besides suppression of central respiratory drive, opioids have been shown in two studies to precipitate upper airway obstruction. Hajiha and colleagues demonstrated that opioids caused a dose-related suppression of tonic brainstem stimulatory input to the genioglossus muscle in rats, a primary muscle involved in upper airway patency. [45] In addition, Montandon and colleagues [18] identified a distinct site of the rat medulla that is associated with opioid-induced suppression of hypoglossal activity. This region is located caudally, dorsally, medially to the pre-BotC, is innervated by pre-BotC neurons, corresponds to the site of hypoglossal premotor neurons identified in neonatal rats in vivo and the parahypoglossal nucleus in adults, and is highly associated with opioid-induced suppression of hypoglossal muscle activity.

Obstructive Sleep Apnea and Chronic Opioid Use

Multiple studies have shown that OSA is highly prevalent among chronic opioid users. [46] [43] [44] Sharkey and colleagues found that OSA (35.2%) was more common than CSA (14.1%) in 71 subjects on methadone maintenance treatment for at least 3 months duration. A case control study by Guilleminault and coworkers in 44 chronic opioid users with OSA (mean AHI 43.9 ± 5.2/hour of sleep, AHI – the number of apneas and hypopneas divided by total hours of sleep, normal < 5/hour) reported a high rate of centrals apneas on treatment with CPAP (CAI – central apnea index 13.8 ±2.8/hour of sleep) or bi-level (CAI 11.5 ±2.1/hour of sleep). The authors also found that compared to controls, the obstructive apnea pattern on polysomnograms of chronic opioid users demonstrated a progressive decrease of inspiratory effort (rather than an expected increase in effort) during the apnea. In addition, the mixed apnea (OSA plus CSA) pattern showed unusually long expiratory pauses before an inspiratory effort was initiated. This finding was described in the Montandon et al study [18] in that the reduction in respiratory rate was due to a prolonged expiratory time without change in inspiratory time.

Opioids are known to cause respiratory depression by acting directly on brainstem respiratory centers. Individuals with OSA are at greater risk for potentially fatal opioid-induced respiratory depression, when the drive to breathe is diminished or abolished during sleep. Post-operative OSA patients receiving opioid analgesia have increased post-operative respiratory complications and respiratory arrest. [47] [48] [49]

Potential Mechanisms for CSA with Chronic Opioid Use

CSA associated with chronic opioid use should be differentiated from other types of CSA. Cheyne-Stokes Respiration (CSR) associated with systolic heart failure is characteristic of a smooth and gradual crescendo-decrescendo respiratory pattern with a much longer cycle time. Idiopathic CSA typically shows a male preponderance with significant arousals from sleep. The pathogenesis of CSA associated with chronic opioid use is likely multi-factorial and ~~is~~ related to the interplay between abnormalities of the central controller as well as central and peripheral chemoreception. Opioid blood concentration is the best predictor for the development of CSA in chronic opioid use. [31] In this study, methadone blood concentration was significantly associated with the severity of CSA, however this accounted for only 12% of CSA. A depressed central controller plays a critical role in the genesis of CSA, as shown in neonatal rodent studies involving the pre-BotC. Another important finding is a blunted HCVR and increased HVR. An imbalance in central and peripheral chemosensitivity poses a greater risk for periodic breathing or instability in breathing pattern. An elevated peripheral chemosensitivity (HVR) has been shown to be a predisposing factor for sleep disordered breathing. [50]

Central Sleep Apnea and Chronic Opioid Use

Chronic opioid use is a risk factor for the development of central sleep apnea. Robinson and colleagues showed that hydromorphone increased the frequency of central apneas during sleep. [51] One of the earliest studies of individuals on stable methadone maintenance treatment reported six out of ten subjects had a central apnea index (CAI; number of central apneas per hour of sleep) $\geq$ 5/hour (normal < 5/hour), with three subjects demonstrating periodic breathing. [52] Farney and colleagues [53] reported three patients who developed sleep disordered breathing characterized by ataxic breathing, central apneas, sustained hypoxemia, and unusually prolonged obstructive hypopneas secondary to delayed arousal responses associated with long-term opioid therapy. In a separate study of 50 stable patients on methadone maintenance treatment program, Wang and colleagues [31] noted the onset of central apneas during sleep. Walker and colleagues [54] showed the development of ataxic breathing and central apneas during NREM sleep in 70% of patients chronically using opioids compared to 5% of controls. In this study, there was a dose dependent relationship between morphine dose equivalent and the AHI. Ninety-two percent of patients who were on a morphine dose equivalent to > 200 mg had central sleep apnea. In one case report, successful withdrawal of methadone completely resolved sleep disordered breathing in addition to improving daytime sleepiness. [55]

MANAGEMENT OF OPIOID ASSOCIATED SLEEP DISORDERED BREATHING

There is no clear consensus on the treatment of sleep disordered breathing associated with chronic opioid use. Along the same lines, optimal treatment modalities for sleep disordered breathing in chronic opioid users have not been established. In general, the lowest dose of opioids that is effective for pain control is recommended and should be continually monitored for requirement changes. Enrollment in addiction programs or utilizing a multidisciplinary pain management program should be considered.

Noninvasive positive airway pressure (PAP) devices such as CPAP (continuous PAP) or bi-level have been used for the treatment of CSA in chronic opioid users with disappointing results. [56] [57] [58] [59] [60] CPAP provides continuous pressure delivery while bi-level provides constant inspiratory and expiratory pressures throughout the respiratory cycle. CPAP and bi-level effectively treat OSA by relieving upper airway obstruction, but do not treat the central apneas secondary to opioid-induced respiratory depression, and may actually increase the frequency of central apneas [58].

On the other hand, bi-level with back-up respiratory rate (i.e. bi-level S/T) has been shown to be effective. Alattar and Scharf reported six patients on methadone maintenance that had central apneas on polysomnography (total AHI range 28.4-106 with > 50% comprised of central apneas) whom improved on bi-level therapy with back-up respiratory rate. [61] A case control study in 44 chronic opioid users with OSA (mean AHI 43.9 ± 5.2/hour) but without CSA on baseline polysomnogram (mean CAI 0.6 ± 1.4/hour) reported a high rate of development of centrals apneas when treatment with CPAP (CAI 13.8 ±2.8/hour) or bi-level (CAI 11.5 ±2.1/hour) was initiated. [58] However, bi-level with back-up respiratory rate effectively eliminated central apneas (CAI 1.7/hour) as well as obstructive apneas and nocturnal oxygen desaturations, and improved subjective daytime sleepiness. [58]

Adapt servoventilation or ASV (VPAP Adapt SV, ResMed Corp) is a positive airway pressure device much different from CPAP or bi-level. Traditionally, ASV was developed and intended for use with Cheyne-Stokes respiration associated with systolic heart failure. [62] With the Adapt SV, end expiratory pressure (EEP) is set at the level of CPAP to eliminate obstructive apneas. The device continually analyzes minute ventilation and adjusts pressure support plus respiratory rate with each respiratory cycle, with a goal of bringing minute ventilation towards 90% of measured mean, effectively treating the high loop gain (i.e. Loop Gain > 1) associated with Cheyne-Stokes Respiration. The algorithm of the Adapt SV allows an increase in pressure support (above EEP) during hypopneas and reduces pressure support during hyperventilation. In addition, the back-up rate is available to treat central apneas. The device is able to treat obstructive apneas, hypopneas, and central apneas.

Since development it has been used with increasing popularity for various types of sleep disordered breathing including treatment-emergent central apneas (i.e. Complex Apnea Syndrome) and most recently, central apneas associated with chronic opioid use. Farney and colleagues attempted the use of ASV in the treatment of 22 sleep disordered breathing in patients who chronically use opioids with disappointing results. [60] This may have been secondary to persistence of obstructive / hypopnea events from ineffective application of end expiratory pressure during the study. In this study, the end-expiratory pressure (EEP) was set at 5 cm H_2O and was not titrated. With EEP set at 5 cm H_2O, it is likely below the pressure required to maintain airway patency (therefore obstructive events persisted). Two studies have shown promising results with the ASV in chronic opioid induced CSA. [59] [57] Javaheri consecutively evaluated five patients with OSA on chronic opioid therapy and found that ASV effectively eliminated central apneas (average AHI decreased from 70 to 20, with a CAI of 0). In this study, EEP was adjusted to effectively eliminate obstructive events. End expiratory pressure (EEP) titration with appropriate adjustment of both inspiratory and expiratory pressures is necessary when treating combined OSA and CSA. Further studies are needed to better understand the most effective positive airway pressure delivery for the treatment CSA in chronic opioid users.

Conclusion

It is important to understand the effects of chronic opioid use on the sleeping patient, and how to approach sleep disordered breathing that combine elements of both upper airway obstruction and suppression of central respiratory drive. Sleep disordered breathing associated with chronic opioid use is under-recognized and under-appreciated by healthcare professionals. Given the disruption of sleep architecture, increased incidence of sleep disordered breathing, increased morbidity and mortality associated with long-term opioid therapy, diagnosis and institution of appropriate therapy in these patients are warranted. Longitudinal, prospective studies of patients with chronic opioid use are needed to assess the long-term effects and on clinical outcomes including morbidity, mortality, and overall quality of life.

The authors declared no conflict of interests.

References

[1] Relieving Pain in America. Institute of Medicine of the National Academies; 2011.

[2] Joranson DE, Ryan KM, Gilson AM, Dahl JL. Trends in medical use and abuse of opioid analgesics. *JAMA* 2000; 283: 1710-1714.

[3] ARCOS. Automation of Reports and Consolidated Orders System. Retail drug summary. In: US Department of Justice DEA (ed). 2005.

[4] The TEDS Report, Changing Substance Abuse Patterns among Older Admissions. SAMHSA; 1992-2008.

[5] Monitoring the future (MTF) survey, US. In: Services DoHaH (ed). 2005.

[6] Unintentional Drug Poisoning in the United States. In: National Center for Injury Prevention and Control CfDCaP (ed). 2010.

[7] Increase in poisoning deaths caused by non-illicit drugs - Utah, 1991 - 2003. *MMWR Morb Mortal Wkly Rep* 2005; 54: 33-36.

[8] Shook JE, Watkins WD, Camporesi EM. Differential roles of opioid receptors in respiration, respiratory disease, and opiate-induced respiratory depression. *Am. Rev. Respir Dis.* 1990; 142: 895-909.

[9] Pattinson KT. Opioids and the control of respiration. *Br. J. Anaesth.* 2008; 100: 747-758.

[10] Smith JC, Ellenberger HH, Ballanyi K, Richter DW, Feldman JL. Pre-Botzinger complex: a brainstem region that may generate respiratory rhythm in mammals. *Science* 1991; 254: 726-729.

[11] Feldman JL, Del Negro CA. Looking for inspiration: new perspectives on respiratory rhythm. *Nat. Rev. Neurosci.* 2006; 7: 232-242.

[12] Janczewski WA, Feldman JL. Distinct rhythm generators for inspiration and expiration in the juvenile rat. *J. Physiol.* 2006; 570: 407-420.

[13] Mellen NM, Janczewski WA, Bocchiaro CM, Feldman JL. Opioid-induced quantal slowing reveals dual networks for respiratory rhythm generation. *Neuron* 2003; 37: 821-826.

[14] Gray PA, Rekling JC, Bocchiaro CM, Feldman JL. Modulation of respiratory frequency by peptidergic input to rhythmogenic neurons in the preBotzinger complex. *Science* 1999; 286: 1566-1568.

[15] Gray PA, Janczewski WA, Mellen N, McCrimmon DR, Feldman JL. Normal breathing requires preBotzinger complex neurokinin-1 receptor-expressing neurons. *Nat. Neurosci.* 2001; 4: 927-930.

[16] McKay LC, Janczewski WA, Feldman JL. Sleep-disordered breathing after targeted ablation of preBotzinger complex neurons. *Nat. Neurosci.* 2005; 8: 1142-1144.

[17] McKay LC, Feldman JL. Unilateral ablation of pre-Botzinger complex disrupts breathing during sleep but not wakefulness. *Am. J. Respir. Crit. Care Med.* 2008; 178: 89-95.

[18] Montandon G, Qin W, Liu H, Ren J, Greer JJ, Horner RL. PreBotzinger complex neurokinin-1 receptor-expressing neurons mediate opioid-induced respiratory depression. *J. Neurosci*; 31: 1292-1301.

[19] Santiago TV, Edelman NH. Opioids and breathing. *J. Appl. Physiol.* 1985; 59: 1675-1685.

[20] Lahiri S, Roy A, Baby SM, Hoshi T, Semenza GL, Prabhakar NR. Oxygen sensing in the body. *Prog. Biophys. Mol. Biol.* 2006; 91: 249-286.

[21] Dahan A, Nieuwenhuijs D, Teppema L. Plasticity of central chemoreceptors: effect of bilateral carotid body resection on central CO2 sensitivity. *PLoS Med.* 2007; 4: e239.

[22] Wood JB, Frankland AW, Eastcott HH. Bilateral removal of carotid bodies for asthma. *Thorax* 1965; 20: 570-573.

[23] Holton P, Wood JB. The effects of bilateral removal of the carotid bodies and denervation of the carotid sinuses in two human subjects. *J. Physiol.* 1965; 181: 365-378.

[24] Weil JV, McCullough RE, Kline JS, Sodal IE. Diminished ventilatory response to hypoxia and hypercapnia after morphine in normal man. *N. Engl. J. Med.* 1975; 292: 1103-1106.

[25] Sarton E, Olofsen E, Romberg R, den Hartigh J, Kest B, Nieuwenhuijs D *et al.* Sex differences in morphine analgesia: an experimental study in healthy volunteers. *Anesthesiology* 2000; 93: 1245-1254; discussion 1246A.

[26] Bailey PL, Lu JK, Pace NL, Orr JA, White JL, Hamber EA *et al.* Effects of intrathecal morphine on the ventilatory response to hypoxia. *N. Engl. J. Med.* 2000; 343: 1228-1234.

[27] Poole SL, Deuchars J, Lewis DI, Deuchars SA. Subdivision-specific responses of neurons in the nucleus of the tractus solitarius to activation of mu-opioid receptors in the rat. *J. Neurophysiol.* 2007; 98: 3060-3071.
[28] Wang D, Teichtahl H. Opioids, sleep architecture and sleep-disordered breathing. *Sleep Med. Rev.* 2007; 11: 35-46.
[29] Banzett RB, Adams L, O'Donnell CR, Gilman SA, Lansing RW, Schwartzstein RM. Using Laboratory Models to Test Treatment: Morphine Reduces Dyspnea and Hypercapnic Ventilatory Response. *Am. J. Respir. Crit. Care Med.* 2011.
[30] Teichtahl H, Wang D, Cunnington D, Quinnell T, Tran H, Kronborg I *et al.* Ventilatory responses to hypoxia and hypercapnia in stable methadone maintenance treatment patients. *Chest* 2005; 128: 1339-1347.
[31] Wang D, Teichtahl H, Drummer O, Goodman C, Cherry G, Cunnington D *et al.* Central sleep apnea in stable methadone maintenance treatment patients. *Chest* 2005; 128: 1348-1356.
[32] Wijdicks EF. Biot's breathing. *J. Neurol Neurosurg Psychiatry* 2007; 78: 512-513.
[33] Quaranta AJ, D'Alonzo GE, Krachman SL. Cheyne-Stokes respiration during sleep in congestive heart failure. *Chest* 1997; 111: 467-473.
[34] Dimsdale JE, Norman D, DeJardin D, Wallace MS. The effect of opioids on sleep architecture. *J. Clin. Sleep Med.* 2007; 3: 33-36.
[35] Shaw IR, Lavigne G, Mayer P, Choiniere M. Acute intravenous administration of morphine perturbs sleep architecture in healthy pain-free young adults: a preliminary study. *Sleep* 2005; 28: 677-682.
[36] Bernards CM, Knowlton SL, Schmidt DF, DePaso WJ, Lee MK, McDonald SB *et al.* Respiratory and sleep effects of remifentanil in volunteers with moderate obstructive sleep apnea. *Anesthesiology* 2009; 110: 41-49.
[37] Kay DC. Human sleep during chronic morphine intoxication. *Psychopharmacologia* 1975; 44: 117-124.
[38] Kay DC. Human sleep and EEG through a cycle of methadone dependence. *Electroencephalogr Clin. Neurophysiol.* 1975; 38: 35-43.
[39] Martin WR, Jasinski DR, Haertzen CA, Kay DC, Jones BE, Mansky PA *et al.* Methadone--a reevaluation. *Arch. Gen. Psychiatry,* 1973; 28: 286-295.
[40] Howe RC, Hegge FW, Phillips JL. Acute heroin abstinence in man: II. Alterations in rapid eye movement (REM) sleep. *Drug Alcohol Depend* 1980; 6: 149-161.
[41] Howe RC, Hegge FW, Phillips JL. Acute heroin abstinence in man: I. Changes in behavior and sleep. *Drug Alcohol Depend* 1980; 5: 341-356.
[42] Howe RC, Phillips JL, Hegge FW. Acute heroin abstinence in man. III. Effect upon waking and slow wave sleep. *Drug Alcohol Depend* 1980; 6: 247-262.
[43] Mogri M, Desai H, Webster L, Grant BJ, Mador MJ. Hypoxemia in patients on chronic opiate therapy with and without sleep apnea. *Sleep Breath* 2009; 13: 49-57.
[44] Webster LR, Choi Y, Desai H, Webster L, Grant BJ. Sleep-disordered breathing and chronic opioid therapy. *Pain Med.* 2008; 9: 425-432.
[45] Hajiha M, DuBord MA, Liu H, Horner RL. Opioid receptor mechanisms at the hypoglossal motor pool and effects on tongue muscle activity in vivo. *J. Physiol.* 2009; 587: 2677-2692.

[46] Sharkey KM, Kurth ME, Anderson BJ, Corso RP, Millman RP, Stein MD. Obstructive sleep apnea is more common than central sleep apnea in methadone maintenance patients with subjective sleep complaints. *Drug Alcohol Depend*; 108: 77-83.

[47] Catley DM, Thornton C, Jordan C, Lehane JR, Royston D, Jones JG. Pronounced, episodic oxygen desaturation in the postoperative period: its association with ventilatory pattern and analgesic regimen. *Anesthesiology* 1985; 63: 20-28.

[48] Ostermeier AM, Roizen MF, Hautkappe M, Klock PA, Klafta JM. Three sudden postoperative respiratory arrests associated with epidural opioids in patients with sleep apnea. *Anesth Analg.* 1997; 85: 452-460.

[49] Esclamado RM, Glenn MG, McCulloch TM, Cummings CW. Perioperative complications and risk factors in the surgical treatment of obstructive sleep apnea syndrome. *Laryngoscope* 1989; 99: 1125-1129.

[50] Dunai J, Kleiman J, Trinder J. Ventilatory instability during sleep onset in individuals with high peripheral chemosensitivity. *J. Appl. Physiol.* 1999; 87: 661-672.

[51] Robinson RW, Zwillich CW, Bixler EO, Cadieux RJ, Kales A, White DP. Effects of oral narcotics on sleep-disordered breathing in healthy adults. *Chest* 1987; 91: 197-203.

[52] Teichtahl H, Prodromidis A, Miller B, Cherry G, Kronborg I. Sleep-disordered breathing in stable methadone programme patients: a pilot study. *Addiction* 2001; 96: 395-403.

[53] Farney RJ, Walker JM, Cloward TV, Rhondeau S. Sleep-disordered breathing associated with long-term opioid therapy. *Chest* 2003; 123: 632-639.

[54] Walker JM, Farney RJ, Rhondeau SM, Boyle KM, Valentine K, Cloward TV *et al.* Chronic opioid use is a risk factor for the development of central sleep apnea and ataxic breathing. *J. Clin. Sleep Med.* 2007; 3: 455-461.

[55] Ramar K. Reversal of sleep-disordered breathing with opioid withdrawal. *Pain Pract.* 2009; 9: 394-398.

[56] Morgenthaler TI, Gay PC, Gordon N, Brown LK. Adaptive servoventilation versus noninvasive positive pressure ventilation for central, mixed, and complex sleep apnea syndromes. *Sleep* 2007; 30: 468-475.

[57] Allam JS, Olson EJ, Gay PC, Morgenthaler TI. Efficacy of adaptive servoventilation in treatment of complex and central sleep apnea syndromes. *Chest* 2007; 132: 1839-1846.

[58] Guilleminault C, Cao M, Yue HJ, Chawla P. Obstructive sleep apnea and chronic opioid use. *Lung*; 188: 459-468.

[59] Javaheri S, Malik A, Smith J, Chung E. Adaptive pressure support servoventilation: a novel treatment for sleep apnea associated with use of opioids. *J. Clin. Sleep Med.* 2008; 4: 305-310.

[60] Farney RJ, Walker JM, Boyle KM, Cloward TV, Shilling KC. Adaptive servoventilation (ASV) in patients with sleep disordered breathing associated with chronic opioid medications for non-malignant pain. *J. Clin. Sleep Med.* 2008; 4: 311-319.

[61] Alattar MA, Scharf SM. Opioid-associated central sleep apnea: a case series. *Sleep Breath* 2009; 13: 201-206.

[62] Teschler H, Dohring J, Wang YM, Berthon-Jones M. Adaptive pressure support servo-ventilation: a novel treatment for Cheyne-Stokes respiration in heart failure. *Am. J. Respir. Crit. Care Med.* 2001; 164: 614-619.

In: Opioids: Pharmacology, Clinical Uses and Adverse Effects ISBN 978-1-61942-101-1
Editors: Djavakhi Tvildiani and Kakha Gegechkori

Chapter 2

PAIN CONCEPTS AND TREATMENT BY OPIOIDS: HISTORIC REVIEW

Merab G. Tsagareli
Ivane Beritashvili Institute of Physiology,
Tbilisi, Georgia

ABSTRACT

Even though we already know from physiological studies that special receptors are responsible for conducting pain sensations to the brain, the phenomenon of pain still remains a medical and social problem. For centuries, physicians were helpless in the battle against pain. They could ease pain sensations with a few drugs, but they could not eliminate it. However, humankind struggled against pain from the very beginning, for thousands of years. As time went on, he used of medicinal herbs in the form of soporific sponges, opium juices and extracts from henbane. Particularly, at the close of the Middle Ages doctors had learnt to put their patients to sleep with pan relieving extracts obtained from the root and fruits mandrake, one of the oldest medicinal plants known to man, also known as mandragora. But until the 19th century pharmacy did not have some sort of effective drugs for pain relief. As early as 1806, the German pharmacist F.W. Sertürner succeeded in deriving an alkaloid from opium for the fight against pain, which he called "morphine", after the Greek god Morpheus. This was a reversion to the antique origins of medicine, in existence at the time of Hippocrates and his medical school, the juice of the poppy, opium were used for relieve pain, fever and insomnia. Knowledge of this drug, which in Greece and the Middles East was easy to obtain from the poppy, remained in use in popular medicine for centuries. This article provides historical perspective on pain concepts and evolution of pain therapy.

Keywords: Algesia, analgesia, anti-nociception, nociceptors, history of medicine, pain therapy.

Introduction

Pain is the oldest medical problem and the universal physical affliction of humankind, yet it has been little understood in physiology until very recently. The philosophical, political, ethnical and religious meanings of pain defined the suffering of individuals for much of human history. We talk about pain as though we are all talking about the same thing. Yet history reveals pain is different for every person who experiences it, and understood differently in different times and epochs, nations and places. Various eras and cultures emphasize different aspects of pain. Clearly, our understanding of pain, and how we treat it, is subject to the ideas, cultural and historical norms of the era and culture in which we live/are situated. Obviously, early humans related pain to evil, magic, and demons. Relief of pain was the responsibility of sorcerers, shamans, priests, and priestesses, who used herbs, rites, and ceremonies as their treatments.

In western civilization, pain is generally agreed-upon as an experience, which involves more than just physical sensations (Mann, 1988; Morris, 1991). It is now recognized that pain, particularly chronic pain, involves a combination of physiological and psychological factors, i.e. thoughts and feelings as well as neurological factors, e.g. changes in patterns of neuronal firing. However, this understanding is relatively new, and marks a significant break with tradition; for the last 300 years, up until about 30 years ago, pain was primarily thought of as a physical problem (Meldrum, 2003; Rey, 1998).

Today, even though we already know from physiological study that special receptors (nociceptors) are responsible for conducting pain sensations to the brain through the body's central nervous system, the phenomenon of pain still remains a puzzle. On the one hand, it warns and protects us, on the other hand, it torments us and can drive us the deepest despair (Fields, 1987; Melzack, 1973; Wall, Jones, 1991).

With the establishment of Western medicine by Hippocrates and his followers in the fourth century BC did physicians residing near the shrines dedicated to Aesculapius, the god of healing, attempt to define the phenomenon of pain, investigate it rationally and try to eliminate its causes to relieve suffering. Although no effective means were yet available, it was the fundamental principle of Hippocratic medicine that medical treatment should avoid unnecessary pain (Porter, 1997).

This brief review is an attempt to give a general idea of the long periods of time that were necessary during the course of thousands years before pain came to be understood in its full implications, freed from mystical and religious notions, investigated and finally successfully treated.

Pain Concepts in Greco-Roman Antiquity

A few Greek philosophers, such as Alkmaeon, Anaxagoras, Hippocrates and Pythagoras in antiquity, had promoted the idea that the brain was the seat of human sensation and perception. Alkmaeon (ca 500 BC), based on anatomical evidence, first proposed that brain is essential for perception. Although no writings of Alkmaeon survived, it was probably via a fortuitous linkage that his idea of the mental primacy of the brain was transmitted to, and preserved within, the teaching of the Hippocratic School. However, their views did not replace Aristotle's postulate of the heart being the center for sensation and emotions until Renaissance. Nothing, of course, was secure as to mechanisms, two millennia unfolding until the search for mind passed from the ventricles to the cerebral cortex. Nonetheless, Alkmaeon was the beginning, and the ensuing understanding that he initiated is still transforming humanity's perception of natural world, and their place within it (Doty, 2007).

When scanning quite length period from Homer's time (ca 8th century BC) to that of the *Hippocratic Collection,* containing 60 medical texts by Hippocrates and his pupils (430-380 BC), it would be dangerous to try to extent some constant factors or a uniformity of practice in the answers to pain in Greek society. It is possible to go back and discover attitudes, which endured, however, such as the acceptance of pain as an inevitable fact of life for both the ill and healthy alike. The rationalization of illness and pain in the Hippocratic work, which is made by a reinterpretation of symptoms, preserves both the word of patient and the unique relationship he has with the physician. The widespread dissemination of Hippocratic ideas, whose original source had not been Athens, continued the Greek cities of Asia Minor and Alexandria's conquests, to the entire known world (Rey, 1998).

It is very interesting that in five Hippocratic texts the word "anesthesia" appears 12 times to describe loss of sensation by a disease process. The word "analgesia" is related to "anesthesia" for the first time, when it is pointed out that an unconscious patient is insensitive to pain. Hippocrates and his followers rationalized pain as a clinical variable and as a valuable diagnostic and prognostic tool. They used expressive and precise adjectives and well-defined characteristics of pain, such as location, duration, or relation to other symptoms, to elucidate a disease process. They also had a wide terminology for the various types of pain, still in use today. Many cures were described for the treatment of pain, including incisions, effusions, venesection, purges, cauterization and, most interestingly, the use of many plants, such as opium or the application of soporific substances. In particular, Hippocrates refers to opium poppy as "sleep inducing." (Astyrakaki et al. 2010).

Alexandrian physician Herophylus (320-260 BC) gained the information on the brain and the nerves represented real progress in relation to the work of his predecessors. While Aristotle had considered the brain to be a simple cooling organ – designed to regulate the heart action and to induce sleep – when Herophylus became interested in the brain's anatomy, he was able to distinguish the ventricles, and he conferred a particularly important role of on cerebellum in controlling voluntary movements.

The second Greek physician Erasistratus (304-245 BC), originally from Antioch in Syria, studied medicine in Athens and in Cos under the tutelage of Praxagoras before going on to Alexandria. Herophylus and Erasistratus explored a great many others aspects of medicine – including studying the pulse – and they used human dissection as the basis of their anatomical knowledge for an understanding of the nervous system. They prepared the way for Galen's (129-199 AD) work almost four centuries later.

Roman physician Celsus (25 BC–50 AD) lived during the reign of Tiberius in the first century AD. His work illustrates an entirely different aspect of medicine. His scientific view was much more closely allied to the Hippocratic School as it regarding pain as an important clue for prognostic purposes. His *De Re Medicina* is one of the most precious documents in the medicine of Antiquity, giving lengthy explanation about pain.

Claudius Galen (129-199 AD) got his professional successes in Rome where he lived intermittently most his life and was the physician of five Roman emperors, such as Marcus Aurelius, Commodus, and Septimius Severus among others. He has a very special place in ancient medical history. Galen placed considerable importance on pain in his writings, not only as a symptom, but also in his analysis of mechanisms at work in sensation and perception. He associated pain specifically with the general category of touch, the sense responsible for tactile and thermal impressions when the external stimulations or irritations were moderate intensity, and for painful impressions when these contained an element of violence (Rey, 1998).

Since ancient times, man has tried to combat pain with natural healing methods. Therapeutic options for all types of pain ranged from suggestive methods, dietetic procedures and herbal therapies to fasting, balneotherapy, and the mud baths from the Stone Age to great civilizations 5.000 years BC. Not only prehistoric healers and high priest physicians of the Babylonian civilization in Mesopotamia acquired the knowledge and trust in the body's instinctive wisdom, obtained from experience, the legendary Greek Hippocrates with his medical school did so too, by trying to strengthen their patient's natural defenses.

In the ancient Greek temples dedicated to Aesculapius, 400 years BC healers working in a sanatorium-like atmosphere attempted to dispel the fear and pain of those seeking a cure by performing religious rituals such as prayers of supplication, sacrifices, ablutions or processions through the sacred precincts. One of the main therapeutic approaches favored by the disciples of Aesculapius was at least to put patients into a healing sleep by administering extracts of medicinal herbs and executing suggestive rituals. Physicians had learnt to put their patients to sleep with pain-relieving extracts of mandrake, one of the oldest medicinal plants known to man, or using "soporific sponges". Pain-relieving extracts were obtained from the root and the fruits of mandrake (*Mandragora officinarium*), also known as mandragora and the sponges were saturated with extracts of henbane (*Hyosciamus niger*), mandragora roots, hemlock (*Conium maculatum*) and the juice of the poppy (*Papaver somniferum*) (Murken, 2005).

Ancient Healing Methods against Pain in Far East: Traditional Chinese Medicine

Since the end of the twentieth century, more and more traditional natural and alternative healing methods from the Far East are being focused on as therapy for chronic ailments and pain. The reason for this growing acceptance lies, above all, in the fact that the person as a whole is considered in this therapeutic concept, in all his physical and psychological complexity and individuality. Their roots can be traced back to the advanced civilizations of China, Japan, and India, and are over two thousand years old. A further advantage of these alternative healing methods can also be seen in their intuitive, psychosomatic concept takes psychological and spiritual factors that have a crucial influence on pain into consideration. It has been shown, especially in pain therapy, how very successful alternative therapy can be, only when used as part of a long-term holistic therapy and individually-targeted healing plan (Murken, 2005).

Eastern traditional healing methods, referred as alternative medicine in the Western World, have grown from a foundation of philosophical traditions, medical hypotheses and practical experience passed down by doctors and healers from generation to generation through the ages, as is the custom in China, Japan and India. They have been practiced and tested by healing men and women for over thousands of years. The central characteristic of these natural healing methods, which consciously include both the irrational and rational, and supernatural, lies in the preservation and in the restoration of the harmony between the body, the soul and the spirit. It can definitely be said that in all long-lived suffering, especially that which includes pain, this is because the harmony has been disturbed.

In terms of cultural history, it is especially interesting in this case to note that the traditional healing methods from the Far East, just as those from ancient Greek medicine, started from the idea of stimulating the natural healing tendencies, the auto-regulatory strengths of the human organism, through careful and gentle practice. For the most part, this is also applies in the treatment of pain which, having existed over a longer period of time, disturbs the psychic balance and becomes an all-controlling stress factor for the patient. These alternative healing methods, which take their treatment concepts from the rhythms of nature and the observation of biological processes, the application of simple healing substances, taken from elements like light, water, massage, and the use of medicinal herbs or meditation, are always the preferred treatment of patients. They resulted in the compliance reduced, stress factors lessened, and the sensitivity to pain alleviated (Murken, 2005).

Acupuncture and Acupressure

In course of civilization, long before modern scientific medicine that has based on the laws of measuring, weighing and counting, as well as on verifiable experiments for about two hundred years, different methods and strategies were developed. The Hippocratic doctors developed their holistically-targeted humoral doctrine based on the principle of the four fluids theory, which they equated with the four elements, the four seasons, the four organs, the liver, the spleen, the black and the yellow gall, and their substances, and their influence on the body. The balance of these fluids, which is disturbed in the case of illness, could again be harmonized according the beliefs of Hippocrates and his school of medicine, if the illness-causing sections were removed from the organism. This was achieved by bleeding, leeching, enemas or inducing vomiting (Rey, 1998).

Point of reference to old Chinese medicine can indeed be found in this ancient humoral doctrine, which apart from developing a complex drug therapy, also developed acupuncture (Latin: 'acus' – the needle, 'pungere' – to prick). According to Chinese impressive teaching theories, two basic forces govern the body, which may be found throughout entire universe: 'yin' and 'yang'. If one of these two polar principles, which western doctors compare to the sympathetic and parasympathetic components of the vegetative (autonomic) nervous system, is too overpowering in the human body, the balance is disturbed the human organism suffers. 'Yin' and 'yang', as complementary forces, are again positioned in relationship to five elements, seasons, effects, and smells, from which phases of change may be derived. All of these are supported by a life force, 'chi', to which they are constantly being subjected. To these are also assigned pairs of organs, whereby organ systems are meant, the corresponding meridians of which are distributed throughout the entire body, from head to feet. Altogether, Chinese medicine is based on twelve main meridians, assigned to organ systems and numerous specific points appear in parallel on both halves of the body. Very differential needle treatments are applied along these meridians, to bring the two flows of energy back into balance. The two streams of energy, 'yin' and 'yang' are either strengthened or subdued as a result. Both are dependent on each other, like heaven and earth, light and darkness, so that a 'yin' organ and 'yang' organ, for example the kidneys and the bladder, from a functional unit (Murken, 2005).

The success of acupuncture treatment for pain can easily be explained in that the needles inserted in certain areas of the skin activate pain-relieve substances. Nowadays scientific opinion theories that nerve receptors stimulated by needle insertion simply pass on the stimulation via nerve impulses and neurotransmitters, such as endorphins, are released. There are also various scientific theories to explain the efficacy of the acupuncture mechanism (Lewith, Vincent, 1996).

Exactly like acupuncture, acupressure comes from the healing repertoire of traditional Chinese medicine, with its holistic health treatment concept of dynamic interaction in the human body. However, because this method does not depend on the insertion of needles, but tries instead, by simply applying "pressure", to influence the functional dynamic sequences in the human organism in their particular paths (meridians), to reduce suffering and pain. For this reason, it is better suited for self-help than acupuncture and is especially effective for acute sudden pain (Lust, 1980).

Ancient Indian Health Philosophy: Ayurveda

The first signs of the Ayurveda philosophy, which go back to Brahma, the Indian God of Creation, probably began in the time from 1200 to 500 BC, in the so-called Veda period. They were written down in the "Veden", the holy books of the Brahmin, in the time between 2000 to 1000 BC. In later collections of medical works in India (Samhita), especially those of the legendary physicians Charaka, Sushruta, and Vagbhata (ca 600 BC), the basic concept of holistic medicine for the entire individual found its classic form as it was passed down from generation to generation in the Indian traditions (Verma, 1995).

In Sanskrit, the old Indian literary language, the term "Ayurveda" means "knowledge of life" ('veda' – knowledge, 'ayu' – life). This philosophy of health works through natural means, as do the medical practice of the antique Greeks and ancient Chinese-Japanese medical theories. For thousands of years, its goal was to stimulate and stabilize the individual's own healing and defense mechanisms. At the same time, chronic pain was also to be prevented and eased. This generally strengthening healing process tries to achieve and maintain a balance between the body, mind and consciousness so these can exist in agreeable, pain-free harmony (Murken, 2005; Verma, 1995).

Similar to that of ancient Greek and Chinese medicine, some speculative and religious aspects of the medical teaching philosophy of Ayurveda are also mixed in with the empirical areas. According to the Ayurveda philosophy, the body consists of six substances: plasma, blood, flesh, bones, bone morrow and reproductive cells. Ayurveda doctrine of harmony between health and illness states that all illness and their symptoms especially that of pain are caused by loss or an abundance of bodily fluids or a malfunction of bodily tissues. It follows that the 'Prana', which is vital life and healing force inherent in both the universe as well as in the human body, and which corresponds to the universal elementary force 'Chi', is disturbed by the pathological imbalance of the 'tridoschas'. The latter is formed from a mixture of the three elementary components, have an effect on the human organism: 'Vata', 'Pitta' and

'Kapha'. They are responsible for the psychosomatic constitution and function of the human body (Murken, 2005, Verma, 1995).

Since almost all-human illnesses are accompanied by pain, the Ayurveda philosophy recommends that the accompanying imbalance of physical and spiritual forces should be combated with gentle, therapeutic methods and remedies. Especially in this way, general ailments and pain can be alleviated. It should be emphasized that some medicinal plants, for example *Rauwolfiae Serpentina* and *Aloe Vera* were used by Ayurveda therapists. They extracted healing substance from the roots of rauwolfia (alkaloids) and from the leaves of the aloe vera plant (Verma, 1995). Moreover, the purification and cleansing treatments recommended by Ayurverdic physicians are also an ancient and valued method; the venerable Greek physician Hippocrates knew of them already and as a result referred to them in his medicinal concept of for bodily fluids, the relationship of which is, in the case of pain, disturbed. In similar way, at the beginning of the Renaissance, Paracelsus (1493-1541) included purging, or evacuation of bowels, in his therapy of pain, which was also based on humoral pathology (Rey, 1998)

In the old Indian medical tradition, pain, in its development and strength of perception, is not only dependent on the individual and his constitution, but also on the rhythm of nature, with its seasonal changes or moon cycles. In these interactions between macro – and microcosmos, between body, mind and conscious, between individuals and society, it is known only too well by the Vaidia, the Ayurvedic physician, that the success or failure of the individual's life plan also plays a role. For instance, the phenomenon of pain may cause existential problems and, on the other hand, chronic pain may lead to failure and depression (Verma, 1995).

Overall, Ayurveda medicine is especially designed to reinforce physical strength and to rejuvenate, as well as to improve psychological and spiritual abilities. In a modern sense, one might say that the immune system is stimulated, and, as a result, pain is reduced. Arguments for the Ayurveda philosophy are especially its gentle methods, and the good relationship between the therapist and the patient, leading to optimal compliance (Murken, 2005).

The Middle Ages in the Orient World and Avicenna

Pain in the Middle Ages had powerful spiritual and religious contexts, but it was also an important academic issue for physicians. It also presented practical challenges, and analysis and alleviation of pain formed an important component of the consolidating field of medicine developing within medieval universities. Opiates were well known among university-trained physicians and apothecaries in the Middle Ages.

Ibn Sina (980-1037) was a famous Persian philosopher and physician. In the West, Ibn Sina is more commonly known by his Latin name Avicenna. Most of his works were written in Arabic, as it was the language of science at that time. Two of his books achieved an international circulation and influence and were translated into Latin, handwritten and reprinted many times after his death. *The Book of Healing* was, principally, Avicenna's interpretation of Aristotelian Philosophy although it also included chapters about metaphysics, psychology and other sciences. *The Canon of Medicine* was Avicenna's account of the sum of medical knowledge from the period in which he attempted to amalgamate the works of the famous Greek physician Galen with known eastern medical practices, especially the work of Al-Razi (835-925). Avicenna also added his own contributions in what became the reference of medicine for almost six centuries (Goodman, 2006).

In the first volume of *The Canon*, Avicenna defines the nature of pain and describes it in five pages. He classifies pain and relates each type to cause. Moreover, Avicenna extended Galen's classification of four types of pain within *The Canon* and categorized 15 types of pain with their causes. Avicenna appeared to appreciate the importance of pain in medical diagnosis and referred to pain as a diagnostic criterion throughout *The Canon.* Avicenna called pain relief 'Taskeen of Pain' that literally means 'making pain quiet'. In modern Arabic language, 'Taskeen' has become the equivalent of 'Analgesia'. Avicenna included a three-page chapter entitled 'Pain Analgesia' in which he suggested that doctors should always seek the cause of pain through proper diagnosis and that treatment of pain should be directed to the cause of the pain (Tashani, Johnson, 2010).

Avicenna referred to 'anesthetics' as 'Mokhader'. Mokhader has a range of meanings including a place of tranquility, especially for women, and a description of an inebriated man. The word Mokhader was in common use before Avicenna's writings to describe a recipe used to dull the sensation. For example, Al-Razi (Rhazes) used opium as 'Mokhader' prior to surgery.

In the fifth volume 'Pharmacopoeia', Avicenna included ice as 'Mokhader' and he also listed a variety of plants with hypnotic, anesthetic and analgesic action including mandragora or nightshade (*Solanum*), opium and henbane (*Hyoscyamus*). Avicenna advocated the use of various recipes of these agents for anesthesia and analgesia before surgery and was aware of the strength and potential toxicity of some of the formulas. Avicenna advised doctors not to use strong analgesics unless it was necessary absolutely. Avicenna appeared to distinguish between drugs that induced sleep and those that helped to "dull the sensation", although he also claimed that anesthetics might relieve pain by inducing sleep (Tashani, Johnson, 2010).

Further research into Avicenna's reasoning behind his classification would be interesting. Particularly, according to him, organs can be either sensitive or non-sensitive. Sensitive organs produce pain sensation if stimulated while non-sensitive organs like the upper part of the stomach may transmit other sensations like the feeling of the "weight of tumor" while no pain sensation is associated with it. Avicenna further explained how movement, bad substances and bloats cause the sensation of pain. Most of these changes lead to a stretch, pressure or distortion of organs and membranes that in turn causes pain. Furthermore, there are very nice views of Avicenna on the brain working. Avicenna agreed with Galen that nerves carried pain sensation to the brain. Galen identified three conditions for pain perception: the organ to receive impression, a connecting passageway and an organizational centre. Avicenna wrote extensively about brain anatomy and its role as a centre for pain sensation. Both Galen and Avicenna believed that the brain was the principal organ for perception of pain (Rey, 1998, Tashani, Johnson, 2010).

Thus in *The Canon* Avicenna challenged Galen's concept of pain. Galen insisted that injuries (breach of continuity) were the only cause of pain. In contrast, Avicenna suggested that the true cause of pain was a change of the physical condition (temperament change) of the organ whether there was an injury present or not. Avicenna also extended Galen's descriptions of 4 to 15 types of pain. It is now well established that there are specialized (tissue injury) receptors (nociceptors) in many different tissues of the body and their activation may lead to the sensation of pain which occurs in the brain. However, recent advances in pain research indicated that while this is enough to explain nociceptive pain, which is a physiological protective mechanism, it does not explain other types of pain such as neuropathic pain. The mechanism of generating inflammatory and neuropathic pain involve changes of nociceptors sensitization, recruitment of new population of previously unresponsive receptors and neural pathways and changes in brain modulation and perception of pain, thus making devising one theory to how pain occurs an unrealistic approach.

PAIN IN THE RENAISSANCE AND CLASSICAL AGE

Few people know that the great Italian painting artist Leonardo da Vinci (1452-1519) studied not only the human body but he tried to understand how the brain works. According to him, the mind had its seat in the third ventricles of the brain that was reached by sensations from the body and from the special sensory organs via the nerves and spinal cord. In drawing of a man with two bodies and two heads, he presented an allegory of pain and pleasure as a unitary concept of polar opposites, according to classical ideas of classical Greek philosopher Plato (428-347 BC). In significant illustrations of da Vinci all sensory organs are connected to the brain, including pain sensation (Clarke, Dewhurst, 1972; Procacci, Maresca, 1998).

Andreas Vesalius (1514-1564) was an anatomist, physician, and author of one of the most influential books on human anatomy *"De Humani Corporis Fabrica"*. He studied detailed the nervous system and brain.

Vesalius defined a nerve as the mode of transmitting sensation and motion and thus refuted his contemporaries' claims that ligaments and tendons were nerve units. He believed that nerves do not originate from the heart, as was the Aristotelian belief, but that nerves stemmed from the brain. Vesalius' most significant contribution to the study of the brain was his trademark illustrations in which he depicts cerebral structures as the corpus callosum, the thalamus, the caudate nucleus, the lenticular nucleus, the globus pallidus, the putamen, the pulvinar, and the cerebral peduncles for the first time. He postulated that pain was a sensation, which reached to the brain by nerves (Tarshis, 1969).

Methods of relieving of pain in the 16th century provided for the management of wounds with salves and other remedies. Hans von Gerstdorff (1455-1529), a physician from Strasburg and was working in the field of as an army surgeon, wrote outstanding book where he referred to ancient authorities such as Galen and Abu al-Qasim Al-Zahrawi (936–1013) known in the West as Albucasis and who was an Andalusian Arab physician. Albucasis is considered the greatest medieval surgeon to have appeared from the Islamic World, and has been described by some as the father of modern surgery. His comprehensive medical texts shaped both Islamic and European surgical procedures up until the Renaissance. His greatest contribution to history is the *Kitab al-Tasrif*, a thirty-volume encyclopedia of medical practices (Ahmad, 2007).

Von Gerstdorff's book contains 25 full-page woodcuts that display the therapeutic methods and tools available at that time. He advised that in caring for the wounded it is essential to pay attention to pain, stating that the caregiver should check to see if there is major pain or swelling and alleviating any pain and soreness (Zimmermann, 2005).

The national medicinal history in Georgia, that is Caucasian Christian country at the crossroad of Europe and Asia, based on the long history and traditions. According to the ancient Greek tragedian Euripides (ca 480-406), Colchis princess and healer Medea knew various medicinal herbs that used for healing and magic. Zaza Panaskerteli-Tsitsishvili (ca 1425-1498) was a 15th-century Georgian prince, politician, and man of letters known for his compendia of medical arts *"Karabadini"* (Book of Medical Treatment). He is described as "the great healer and head of the wise" in a contemporary record. Zaza's Karabadini (ultimately from the Greek graphidion, "booklet") is an original medical treatise dated to c. 1486. It builds upon anonymous Georgian compendia of Galenic medicine, notably the 11th-century *"Ustsoro Karabadini"* (Peerless Handbook) and the 13th-century *"Tsigni Saakimoy"* (Doctoring Book).

The work summarizes the state of medical knowledge in Georgia and neighboring cultures at that time. Panaskerteli was a proponent of rational therapy. He denied the mystical nature of mental illness and attributed them to the pathological processes in the brain (Pitskhelauri, 1975; Shengelia, 1988). He also transcribed a Georgian translation of the doctrines of John Chrysostom (c. 349–407). A century later, Georgian king Davit XI compiled a handbook on medicine called "*Yadigar Daudi"* (Shengelia, 1984).

The great French surgeon of the renaissance period Ambroise Paré (1510-1590) provided detailed descriptions of the pain associated with wounds and surgery, and suggested methods for its relief. He was the first to describe pain from amputated limbs, almost 300 years later named "phantom pain" by Silas W. Mitchell.

Paré was interested in devising better and more efficient methods of pain treatment. He emphasized the potential of drug preparations featuring opium as the main active ingredient. He was also greatly concerned with the treatment of pain induced by surgery, and defined pain treatment as one of the important tasks of the surgeon. One of the most significant observations of Paré was that analgesia during and after surgery reduced various post-operative risks such as inflammation, fever, and gangrene. Another observation by him was that a positive and cooperative attitude on the part of the patient before surgery helped to improve the outcome of the operation, by which he anticipated today's beneficial concepts of pain coping (Poirier, 2005).

In the 17th century, the theory of nervous system function was much promoted by French philosopher and mathematician René Descartes (1596-1650), dramatically changing the prevailing views on pain. Although, he is perhaps best known for the philosophical statement *"Cogito ergo sum"* (I think, therefore I am) he provided new concept of the functional anatomy of the sensory organs and brain in his famous book *"De Homine",* published posthumously (1662).

In this book, Descartes may be appeared as the first analytical scientist in sensory physiology. He described the basic template for the idea of pain as a signal of physical pathology (later "Specificity Theory" of pain) in his definition of pain: *"Fast moving particles of fire the disturbance passes along the nerve filament until it reaches the brain..."* (cited by Procacci, Maresca, 1998).

In his renowned picture, Descartes visualized the transmission of pain signals via the nerves and spinal cord as bell-pull terminating in the brain ventricles and pineal organ (Figure 1). For him, the pineal organ was the tentative locus of the conscious perception of a pain stimulus. Almost in any modern textbook of neuroscience, the same basic types of illustrations are used to explain the conductance pain signals to the brain.

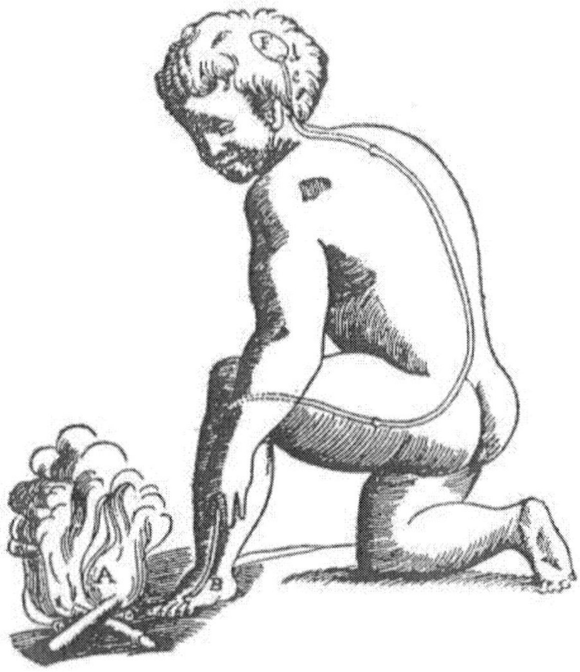

Figure 1. Descartes' drawing of a pathway-oriented pain mechanism. The fire activates pain nerves in the foot of the child and these signals are transmitted via the spinal cord to the brain where they are reflected into motor nerves that draw the foot away from the fire.

While contemplating the mind-body connection, Descartes suggested that sensations stimulated in the body are conveyed directly to the brain, where they are actually perceived. Although this view is now considered overly simplistic, that should not diminish Descartes' insightful realization that sensory perception is in fact a function of the brain. The Cartesian model gave rise to the notion of a "hard-wired system", where pain signals were carried by fixed connections within the nervous system. This idea was reinforced by anatomical studies carried out during the 19th century and has endured, with a few modifications, until fairly recently (Procacci, Maresca, 1992; 1994, Handwerker, 2007). Descartes' ideas were part of a trend toward a more scientific approach to understanding human ills. During the renaissance, greater freedom of thought, increased communication (via the invention of the printing press) and a more secular society, allowed a rational scientific approach to flourish. In the next few hundred years this approach facilitated great advances in understanding and treating pain and disease. Prior to the renaissance, the trend had been to locate the causes of disease outside the body but with the rise of medical science, the causes for pain and illness were increasingly understood in terms of physical injury and thus located inside the body.

The second great figure of the 17th century English scientist and Doctor Thomas Willis (1621-1675) played an important role in history of the nervous system and the brain. He is well known as an author of the discovery the circle of blood vessels that supply the brain with blood (the "Circle of Willis"). He provided overwhelming evidence that the brain substance, including cortex, is the substrate of sensory functions, and not brain ventricles, as previously believed. Moreover, Willis localized the affective dimension of pain in the corpus striatum and corpus callosum. The motor and visceral reflexes associated with pain are initiated here and conducted via the cerebellum and brainstem, whereas the commands for the expression of pain are transmitted to the facial muscles via the pons (Hughes, 1991). It took, thus, 2000 years for Pythagoras's association of pain sensation with the brain to become a generally established concept. English physician Thomas Sydenham (1624-1689) was posthumously known as the "English Hippocrates" and the father of English medicine for his great reformation of medicine in England and as the discoverer of the mechanisms of the spread of disease in epidemic plague. Among his many achievements was the also discovery of a disease, Sydenham's chorea. He promoted the consistent and systematic treatment of pain (Pearce, 1995). Sydenham named the analgesic drug laudanum, a composite of opium, saffron (*Crocus sativus*), cinnamon, and cloves in wine. Based his own experience as a pain patient, he strongly promoted laudanum as an indispensable basic tool of every physician. However, the use opium, consistently promoted by Sydenham, had strong opponents among his contemporaries. One of them was German professor Georg Wolfgang Wedel (1645-1721) who published warnings that, among all medications used by physicians, opium would require the doctor's most serious concern because of its dangerous and potentially lethal effects (Zimmermann, 2005). For thousands of years in the past, up to the beginning of the 20th century, the practice of medicine consisted, for the most part, in the use of extracts and essences from medicinal plants, in addition to psychosomatic medicine and the surgical treatment of external wounds. In this way aromatic oils, extracts or infusions of medicinal herbs such as nettles (*Urtica*), chamomile (*Matricaria*), and juices from the opium during magic rituals were considerably more effective.

In the first century AD, the Roman military physician Pedanius Dioskurides, from Greece, presented an extensive medicinal treasury of over 600 medicinal plants, in which he recommended natural medicine for the treatment of the most prevalent illness. In the middle ages, it was the famous nun, Hildegard von Bingen (1098-1179), an early naturalist, who dedicated her entire life to the study of medicinal herbs. In her theory on natural medicine, she viewed sick people as a physical-spiritual unit, as Hippocrates also did in ancient times, and believed that one must heal them in a comprehensive manner, i.e., in their entirely. Later, in the 16th century a number of noteworthy physicians and pharmacists laid the foundations for today's phytotherapy. Particularly, German Petrus Uffenbach (1566-1635) published a reworked and expanded version of the "Dioskurides" (1610), the German text of which was accompanied by outstanding plant illustrations and explanations. Leonhard Fuchs (1501-1566) pioneered some work before that in extracting medicine from nature with his "New Herbal Book" published in 1543. The medicinal plants mentioned in his textbook were pictured in a very modern and realistic way and explained in great detailed. Finally, Italian Pietro Andrea Matthioli (1501-1577) described 100 new plants and coordinated the medical botany of his time in his *"Discorsi"* ("Commentaries") on the Materia Medica of Dioscurides. The first edition of Mattioli's work appeared in 1544 in Italian and was a further naturopathic compendium (Murken, 2005).

We can say with justification that until the beginning of the synthetic medicines era in the 20th century, the use of various elements of medicinal plants promised the most effective cure. Some of that medicinal plants are still used to pain relieve today, among them Bearberry (*Arctostaphylus uva-ursi*), Chamomile (*Matricaria chamomilla*), Eucalyptus (*E. globulus*), Hawthorn (*Crataegus oxicantha*), Juniper Berry (*J. communis*), Mandrake (*Alraune*), Valerian (*V. officinalis*), Willow (*Salix alba*).

The 19th Century: Great Discoveries in Pain Research

In the 19th century, pain research became a subject of physiological science (Perl, 2007). Swedish Magnus Blix (1849-1904) and German Max von Frey (1852-1932) discovered that the spatial fine structure of cutaneous sensitivity consisted of discrete points at which sensations could be elicited by mechanical, thermal, and/or noxious stimuli. They used calibrated hairs and bristles to exert defined mechanical stimuli to the skin of human subjects. The mosaic of pain points was different from that of touch points. The principal conclusion from these psychophysical experiments was that specific sensory nerve endings exist in the skin for the sensation of painful stimuli. These "pain points" were associated anatomically with the intraepithelial free nerve endings (Zimmermann, 2005).

English Charles S. Sherrington (1857-1952) called a few later, these specific receptors as nociceptors (1903). He used many different styles of experiments to demonstrate that different types of stimulation to a nerve's receptive field led to different responses. Some intense stimuli trigger reflex withdrawal, autonomic responses and pain. By modern definition, a nociceptor is a sensory receptor that responds to potentially damaging stimuli by sending nerve signals to the spinal cord and brain. This process, called nociception, usually causes the perception of pain. An important point for the understanding of the function of nociceptors is that their stimulation threshold is just below tissue-damaging intensity. The function of nociceptors is not to signal existing tissue damage, but to inform the central nervous system when stimuli approach tissue-threatening intensities (Woolf, Ma, 2007).

Von Frey's notions were based on the doctrine of specific nerve energies put forwarded by the German physiologist Johannes Müller (1801–1858) in the first half of the 19th century. The basic proposal of his doctrine is that each sensory modality is the result of the activation of a specific neural system in the brain. If we are able to perceive touch it is because we have a subset of cells in our peripheral and central nervous system that respond to touch. He stated the principle, not before recognized, that the kind of sensation following stimulation of a sensory nerve does not depend on the mode of stimulation but upon the nature of the sense organ. This he termed the "Law of specific energies" of the sense. Von Frey's specificity theory of pain (1895) was a natural development of the Müller's doctrine. He extended Müller's concept to pain sensation, thus reinforcing a strict sensory interpretation of pain (Cervero, 2009).

In contrast, the "intensity theory" or pattern theory of pain represented a development of the Aristotelian concept of pain as a passion of the soul and was articulated in modern form by Adolf Goldscheider (1858-1935) at the turn of the nineteenth century. The basic proposal was that pain is the result of intense stimulation of peripheral receptors, regardless of modality and tissue origin. For the pattern theory, the neural substrate of pain perception consists of sequences of impulses in peripheral and central neurons that lead to pain sensations when certain spatial and temporal patterns of activity are produced (1898). In other words, with increasing intensity of mechanical skin stimulation, the sensations reported by the subjects changed continuously from touch to pain. In Goldscheider view, the neural information for touch and pain originate from the same set of nerve receptors. The emphasis of this interpretation is on patterns of neural activity evoked in the brain by a painful stimulus. According to the modern point of view it is clear that a point has been reached, where neither a strict specificity nor a pattern interpretation can account for all that it is known about pain mechanisms (Cervero, 2009; Zimmermann, 2005).

The Birth of Anesthesia

The first anesthetic effect of nitrous oxide ("laughing gas") was reported as early as 1800 by the English chemist Humphrey Davy (1778-1829), and that substance ether was described in 1818 by the English physicist Michael Faraday (1791-1829). Both of these reports mentioned the possibility that anesthesia could be utilized for surgery. Later, in 1846, John C. Warren (1778-1856) conducted the first surgical operation using ether. The report of Warren's cancer surgery without pain elicited a rush to use ether to prevent pain in various medical conditions. Almost simultaneously, a dentist William T. Morton (1819-1868) used this new type of anesthesia to suppress completely pain sensation during dental extraction. Afterwards, in Edinburgh, James Y. Simpson (1811-1870) used ether in childbirth as early as in 1847. In the same year, he discovered chloroform as an alternative to ether.

Another sensation event, following ether anesthesia was the discovery of local anesthesia by Austrian ophthalmologist Karl Koller (1857-1944) in Vienna. He introduced cocaine, a plant alkaloid extracted from South American coca plants, as a local anesthetic for eye surgery. Prior to this discovery, he had tested solutions such as chloral hydrate and morphine as anesthetics in the eyes of laboratory animals without success. In 1884, Koller demonstrated cocaine's potential as a local anesthetic to the medical community and his findings were a medical breakthrough (Zimmermann, 2005).

Synthesis of Opioid and Non-Opioid Analgesics

Some basic analgesic drugs for systemic (intravenous, intraperitoneal) use were also discovered in the 19th century, like as morphine, aspirin, pyramidon, paracetamol. In 1806, the young German pharmacist Friedrich W. Sertürner (1783-1841) reported on his discovery of the sleep-inducing substance extraction contained in opium. As we mentioned above, the extract of poppy (*Papaver somniferum*) juice extract used in medicine for centuries. He tested this extract in heroic experiments on himself and his friends. However, the publication of his discovery remained unnoticed. After nearly 10 years he resumed his investigation of opium extracts and used the new label 'morphium' (derived from Morpheus, the Greek god of sleep) for sleeping-inducing substance (1817). This publication was widely acknowledged, and Sertürner became famous throughout Europe.

On the other side of the Atlantic, American Civil War imposed great progress in the understanding of pain treatment by opioids and anesthesia. A neurologist Silas Weir Mitchell (1830-1914) provided detailed descriptions of post-traumatic neuralgia, phantom limb pain, and causalgias from cases he treated at the Philadelphia hospital.

In the case of continuous excruciating pain, he routinely administered morphine injections several times a day and reported on the excellent analgesic effects of the morphine. Also interestingly, that Mitchell injected morphine locally to the site of the lesion in case of causalgia and maybe credited him for the first observation of peripheral opioid action. Apart from his good descriptions of the analgesia elicited by morphine treatment, he also reported on very unfavorable physical and moral conditions related to the use of morphine, i.e., the induction of dependence and addiction (Lau, Chung, 2004).

THE 20TH CENTURY: CHALLENGES AND CHANGES IN PAIN CONCEPTS

The first half of the 20th century left millions of people, soldiers and civil patients, in pain from injuries sustained in two world wars. After World War II, anesthesiologists and surgeons were the first to respond to these challenges, resulting in rapidly increasing therapeutic skills and newly developed scientific concepts related to pain. German neurosurgeon Otfried Foerster (1873-1941) was one of the first to use systematically cordotomy (transection of the spinal pathways) for the treatment of pain after World War I. He concluded from some very important clinical observations that spinal sensory transmission is under descending control from the brain (1927).

French surgeon René Leriche (1879-1955) became a provocative and emphatic advocate of pain therapy in France. He coined the concept of pain as a disease to which multiple factors contribute. He emphasized excruciating chronic pain related to dysfunction of the sympathetic nervous system, and therefore he recommended interventions on the sympathetic nervous system. The concepts of pain based on clinical studies by Foerster, Lerich and others were further elaborated by Dutch surgeon and pain theorist William Noordenbos (1910-1990) into a pain theory of central interactions and so by the made a great contribution to the field of pain helped inaugurate the current era of research in pain mechanisms (Noordenbos, 1959).

Furthermore, Swedish neurophysiologist Yngve Zotterman (1892-1982) had recorded the first single nervous impulses (nerve fiber action potentials) in Edgar D. Adrian's (1889-1977) laboratory in Cambridge. Ten years later, he published first action potentials recorded from a single nociceptive nerve fiber (slow nonmyelinated C fiber) in cat's tongue in response to noxious heating (1936).

It was very significant the discovery of Thomas Lewis (1881-1945) who postulated the existence of humoral substances, chemical mediators that slowly increased pain sensitivity in the environment of a primary lesion. Among the mediators, he identified were histamine, bradykinin, and substance P. From these discoveries the concept of neurogenic inflammation emerged, which is now considered to contribute to pain-enhancing interaction between the nervous and immune systems in rheumatic and neurophatic diseases (Lewis, 1942). The American surgeon William K. Livingston (1892-1966) treated and studied complex pain phenomena during World War II, such as referred pain and causalgia, and emphasized their continual exacerbation if they were not treated consistently. He conceptualized the idea on "neuronal pool" of variable excitability in the spinal cord. Livingston began to explore new concepts: the temporal and spatial patterning of pain input, the importance of summation mechanisms, the dynamics of reverberating circuits to account for persistent pain states, and the use of anesthetic blocks and stimulation techniques to modulate pain (Livingston, 1943). His clinical and laboratory experimental observations anticipated many trends in current pain research. These include the role of multiple ascending pathways in pain perception, the powerful influence of descending pain-modulating pathways, the importance of central sensitization, the role of inflammation in activating visceral nociceptors, and the importance of learning, attention, and expectation on perceived pain intensity (Livingston [1965], published posthumously in 1998).

Thus, the concepts developed since 1940s by Livingston and others, relating to spinal mechanisms of hyperalgesia now form a central part of our understanding of the principal components of hyperalgesia and allodynia (pain due to a mechanical stimulus that does not normally provoke pain), and progressive chronicity of pain.

The publication of the "Gate Control" theory of pain by Ronald Melzack and Patrick D. Wall (1925-2001) in 1965 was aimed at an integration of the views of physiology, psychology, and the huge variety of clinical phenomenon related to pain in patients, in an attempt to set up a coherent system of ideas (Figure 2). Particularly, in other words, the gate theory of pain proposed a specific neural mechanism located at the first afferent relay in the spinal cord to illustrate how patterns of impulses in sensory receptors could lead to the modulation of pain sensation (Melzack, Wall, 1965).

The gate theory emphasized the dynamic and plastic components of pain sensations and drew attention to pain modulation as opposed to an interpretation of pain exclusively as an alarm system. It also focused the attention of many investigations on the clinical aspects of pain, away from physiological pain, which contributed a surge of studies on the effects of neuropathic lesions and on the development of animal models of inflammatory and pathological pain (Cervero, 2005). Although some neurophysiological details of the gate control theory were later disproved, this theory provided a new perspective on pain for basic and medical scientist and is now considered the foundation of modern conceptions of pain (Melzack, 1999; Novy, Nelson, 1997).

Nevertheless, the most important milestone in the 20th century probably was the discovery of endogenous opioids (the endorphins, enkephalines, and dynorphines) and the identification of the opioid receptors though which opioid drugs exert their effects, and finally central nervous system descending pain control (modulation) system.

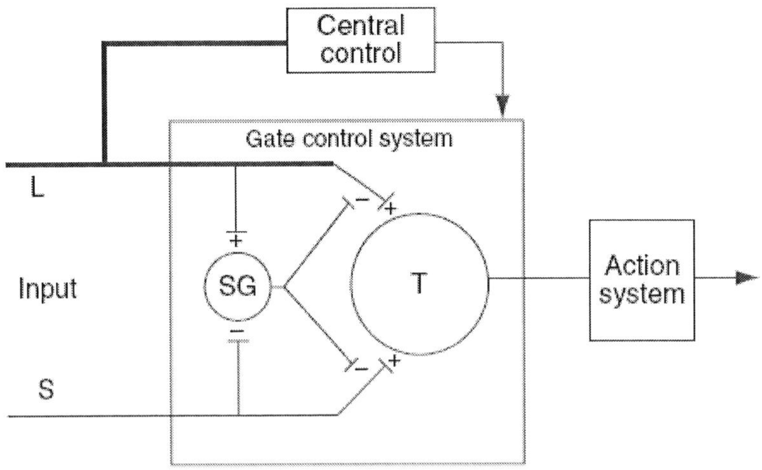

Figure 2. Schematic diagram of the gate theory of pain mechanisms. The diagram shows the presynaptic interaction model between large (L) and small (S) afferent fibers and the key role of spinal cord substantia gelatinosa (SG) neurons controlling the activity of transmission (T) cells, and descending controlling mechanisms of supraspinal structures of the brain.

These findings led to the use of injections of morphine and endorphins, and other opioids, into the cerebrospinal fluid without causing paralysis, numbness, or other severe side effects. This technique is now commonly used in humans to treat pain after surgery and is mainstay for pain relief after caesarean section and other operations in the abdominal and sacral parts of the human body.

CONCLUDING REMARKS

Therapeutic strategies for overcoming pain have developed over thousands of years to an abundance of healing methods, scientific concepts and procedures. They range from aromatherapy as tried and tested in ancient Egypt, Chinese-Japanese traditional medicine, and the Ayurveda healing treatments of India and herbal therapies of the ancient world to the high-tech medicine of the present, with its many disciplines. Astonishingly, since the end of the 20th century, a tendency has been growing more toward the use of these different possibilities, not only as isolated therapeutic procedures, but also in combination, to look at both naturopathic as well as modern standard medicine possibilities for the treatment of pain patients. It is well known today from numerous examinations on pain, its origin, its course and through the methods for its treatment, that in the majority of cases the psychological condition of the pain sufferer is also involved, in some form or other. With the sensation and feeling of pain, the body not only raises an alarm, but the painful sensations also penetrate the psychosomatic core of the person affected.

As the 21st century unfolds, advances in pain research are creating a less grim future and we hope that future that includes a better understanding of pain, along with greatly improved treatments to keep it in check.

REFERENCES

Ahmad Z. (2007) Al-Zahrawi – the father of surgery. *ANZ Journal of Surgery*, 77, Suppl. 1, A83.

Astyrakaki E., Papaioannou A., Askitopoulou H. (2010) References to Anesthesia, Pain, and Analgesia in the Hippocratic Collection. *Anesthesia and Analgesia*, 110(1):188-94.

Cervero F. (2005) The gate theory, then and now. In: *The Path of Pain 1975-2005*, eds. H. Merskey, J.D. Loeser, R. Dubner. Seatle: IASP Press, pp. 33-48.

Cervero F. (2009) Pain theories. In: *Science of Pain*, eds. A.I. Basbaum and M.C. Bushnell, San Diego: Elsevier, pp. 11-42.

Clarke E,, Dewhurst K. (1972) *An illustrated History of Brain Function*. Berkeley: California Univ. Press.

Doty R.W. (2007) Alkmaion's discovery that brain creates mind: a revolution in human knowledge comparable to that of Copernicus and of Darwin. *Neuroscience*, 147:561-568.

Fields H.L. (1987) *Pain*. New York: McGraw-Hill.

Goodman L.E. (2006) *Avicenna*. London: Cornell Univ. Press.

Handwerker H.O. (2007) From Descartes to fMRI. Pain theories and pain concepts. *Schmerz*, 21(4):307-317 (German, English Abstract).

Hughes J.T. (1991) *Thomas Willis (1621-1675): His life and Work*. London: Royal Soc. Med.
Lau F.H., Chung K.C. (2004) Silas Weir Mitchell, MD: the physician who discovered causalgia. *J. Hand Surgery*, 29(2):181-187.
Lewis T. (1942) *Pain*. New York: Macmillan.
Lewith G.T., Vincent C. (1996) On the evaluation of the clinical effects of acupuncture. *J. Altern. Complem. Med.*, 2(1):79-90.
Livingston W.K. (1943) *Pain Mechanisms*. New York: Macmillan.
Livingston W.K. (1998) *Pain and Suffering*, ed. H.L. Fields. Seatle: IASP Press.
Lust B. (1980) *Zone Therapy: Relieving Pain and Sickness by Nerve Pressure*. New York.
Mann R. (1988) *The History of the Management of Pain. From Early Principles to Present Pain*. New York: Parthenon Pub. Group.
Meldrum M.L. (2003) A capsule history of pain management. *J. Am. Med. Assoc.*, 290(18): 2470-2475.
Melzack R. (1973) *The Puzzle of Pain*. Harmoudsworth: Penguin.
Melzack R. (1999) From the gate to the neuromatrix. *Pain*, Suppl. 6: S121-S126.
Melzack R., Wall P.D. (1965) Pain mechanisms: a new theory. *Science*, 150:971-979.
Morris D.B. (1991) *The Culture of Pain*. Los Angeles: California Univ. Press.
Murken A.H. (2005) *Pain as Man's Constant Companion, from Birth to Death*. Vols. 1/2. Herzogenrath: Verlag Murken-Altrogge.
Noordenbos W. (1959) *Pain*. Amsterdam: Elsevier.
Novy D.M., Nelson D.V. (1997) Toward a broader view of the evolution of pain concepts. *Pain Forum*, 6(1):65-67.
Pearce J.M. (1995) Thomas Sydenham "The British Hippocrates". *J. Neurol. Neurosurg. Psychiatry,* 58(3):292.
Perl E.R. (2007) Ideas about pain, a historic view. *Nat. Rev. Neurosci.*, 8(1):71-80.
Pitskhelauri G.Z. (1975) Zaza Panaskerteli-Tsististhvili, Georgian scientist and physician (on the 550th anniversary of birth). *Sov. Zdravookhr.*, No.5:75-78 (in Russian).
Porter R. (1997) *The Greatest Benefit to Mankind: A Medical History from Antiquity to the Present*. London: Harper Collins.
Procacci P., Maresca M. (1992) The concept of pain in the 17th century. *Med. Secoli.*, 4(3):63-70.
Procacci P., Maresca M. (1994) Descartes's physiology of pain. *Pain*, 58(2):133.
Procacci P., Maresca M. (1998) Historical development of the concept of pain. *Pain Clinic*, 10:211-228.
Poirier J.-P. (2005) *Ambroise Paré. Un urgentiste au XVIe siècle*. Paris: Pygmalion.
Rey R. (1998) *The History of Pain*. Cambridge, MA: Harward Univ. Press.
Shengelia M.S. (1984) *History of Georgian Medicine*. 2ed ed., Tbilisi: Ganatleba (in Russian).
Shengelia M.S. (1988) *Zaza Panaskerteli-Tsistishvili*. 2ed ed., Tbilisi: Sabchota Sakartvelo (in Russian).
Tarshis J. (1969) *Andreas Vesalius, Father of Modern Anatomy*. New York: The Dial Press Inc.
Tashani O.A., Johnson M.I. (2010) Avicenna's concept of pain. *Libyan J. Med.*, 5: 5253-5256.
Verma V. (1995) *Ayurveda: A Way of Life*. Boston, MA: Weiser Books.

Wall P.D., Jones M. (1991) *Defeatin Pain: The War Against Silent Epidemic*. New York: Plenum.

Woolf CJ., Ma Q. (2007) Nociceptors – Noxious stimulus detectors. *Neuron*, 55:353-364.

Zimmermann M. (2005) The history of pain concepts and treatment before IASP. In: *The Path of Pain 1975-2005*, eds. H. Merskey, J.D. Loeser, R. Dubner. Seatle: IASP Press, pp. 1-21.

In: Opioids: Pharmacology, Clinical Uses and Adverse Effects ISBN 978-1-61942-101-1
Editors: Djavakhi Tvildiani and Kakha Gegechkori

Chapter 3

µ-Opioid Receptor Modulation of Oxytocin and Vasopressin Release in the Hypothalamic-Neurohypophysial System

José R. Lemos[1], Govindan Dayanithi[2], G. Taimur Dad[1], Edward E. Custer[1], and Sonia Ortiz-Miranda[1]*

[1]Department of Microbiology and Physiological Systems, University of Massachusetts School of Medicine, Worcester, MA, US

[2]Institute of Experimental Medicine, Department of Cellular Neurophysiology, Academy of Sciences of the Czech Republic, EU Research Centre of Excellence, Prague; Czech Republic

Abstract

The Hypothalamic-Neurohypophysial System (HNS) in mammals controls diuresis and parturition through the release of the neuropeptides arginine-vasopressin (AVP) and oxytocin (OT). These neuropeptides are synthesized in hypothalamic Magnocellular neurons (MCNs) and are secreted into the blood stream from terminals in the neurohypophysis (NH). Neuroendocrine function in the HNS is modulated by opioids, either released endogenously or applied exogenously, by acting on µ- or κ-selective opioid receptors. Parturition is disrupted and the milk ejection reflex is inhibited during lactation when OT release is interrupted by opiate drugs. Also, water and salt balance are regulated by centrally or peripherally administered opioids acting on the HNS.

Mu- and kappa- opioid receptors have been identified in the soma and nerve endings of MCN using pharmacological and autoradiographic techniques. When activated in NH terminals, opioid receptors differentially inhibit various types of voltage-gated calcium channels (VGCC), hence modulating the amount of OT and/or AVP being released. In the present research, we characterized the expression of both µ- or κ-opioid receptors and

* Corresponding author: Sonia Ortiz-Miranda, Ph.D., MaPS Department, University of Massachusetts Medical School, 55 Lake Ave North, Worcester, MA 01655. Tel. 508-856-8927 Fax 508-856-5997. E-mail: sonia.ortiz-miranda@umassmed.edu.

VGCCs using immunocytochemical techniques and provide evidence for a differential targeting of channels in OT *vs.* AVP nerve terminals. We propose a model that can explain how opiate effects on VGCCs can directly mediate differences in the control of neurohypophysial OT and/or AVP release.

Keywords: calcium channels, neuropeptides, opioids

Introduction

Opiate Action in the Central Nervous System

The presence of opioid-containing neurons and their projection pathways in the central nervous system (CNS) strongly suggest that neurotransmission is modulated by opioids at diverse sites (Koob, 1992; Leng et al., 1988b; Lewis et al., 1985; Self and Nestler, 1995; Mansour et al., 1995; 1989; Pert et al., 1973). This anatomical evidence is supported by physiological and behavioral evidence of opiate effects within many brain regions (Schoffelmeer and Mulder, 1994; Hughes, et al., 1975). Although there are reports of morphine increasing the spontaneous firing of neurons in the Nucleus Accumbens (Chrobak and Napier, 1993), the net effect of opiate receptor activation is generally an inhibition of firing activity and presumably, a functional reduction in transmitter release (Mansour et al., 1995; Zamponi et al., 1997). Opiates are thus thought to initially affect the brain by influencing the amount of neurotransmitter present at synapses through interactions with specific receptors (Mansour et al., 1989). Whether opiates functionally reduce or increase the effective amount of transmitter release directly (presynaptically) and/or indirectly (postsynaptically) is still an active area of research.

General Physiology of the HNS

Magnocellular neurons in the Paraventricular and Supraoptic nuclei of the hypothalamus project their axons into the neurohypophysis, where they release oxytocin (OT) and vasopressin (AVP) into the blood circulation (Figure 1; reviewed in Lemos, 2001). Each neurohormone regulates various physiological functions (see Leng et al., 1999; Lohmeier, 2003); OT being primarily important in processes related to parturition (Russell et al., 2003) and AVP controlling diuresis (Baylis, 1987; Acher & Chauvet, 2002).

Opioids Effects in the HNS

The initial observations of opiate effects on the HNS were made by DeBodo (1944), who noted that morphine, acting via the CNS system, had an antidiuretic effect in humans. More recent studies on the effects of opiates on plasma concentration of HNS neuropeptide levels, drinking behavior, diuresis, or other relevant parameters have shown that OT and/or AVP secretion is inhibited by opiates (Hartman et al., 1986; 1987; Summy-Long et al., 1984; Oiso et al., 1988; Clarke et al., 1979; Paronis et al., 1995) and that tolerance and dependence develop during chronic opiate administration (Bicknell et al., 1980; Pumford et al., 1991; Leng et al., 1989; Russell et al., 1995). However, other studies have shown different and even

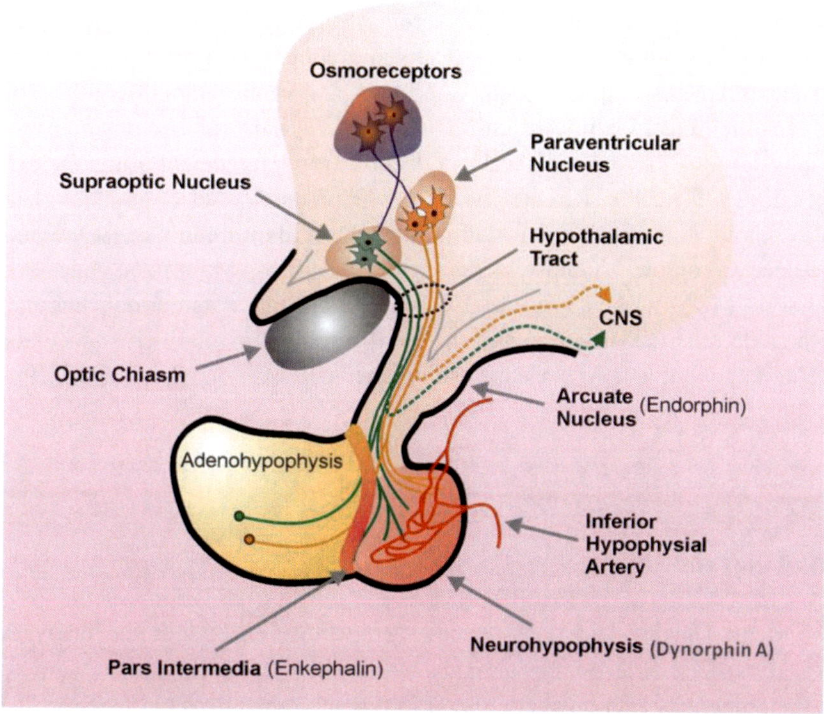

Figure 1. Schematic drawing showing the general anatomy of the HNS. Magnocellular neurons in the Supraoptic and Paraventricular nuclei, synthesizing AVP and OT, project their axons to the posterior pituitary gland as well as to other CNS targets. The local endogenous release of opioids, either from the Arcuate nucleus, Pars Intermedia or the Neurohypophysis itself is highlighted. (Modified from Lemos, 2001).

opposite effects (Nordmann et al., 1986). In addition to these effects, a tonic opioid input into oxytocinergic MCNs has been inferred, since in late pregnancy, as well as during lactation, the opiate antagonist naloxone, increases the plasma concentration of OT (but not AVP), accelerating parturition. Moreover, it is well documented that morphine administration slows parturition (Bicknell et al., 1980; Hartman et al., 1986, 1987; Leng et al., 1985, 1987 and1988b). Thus, the question arises as to how morphine can differentially affect parturition and diuresis in this physiological system.

In the hypothalamus, opioids affect the electrical behavior of MCNs, reducing their firing rate and consequently reducing the systemic secretion of OT and AVP from the neurohypophysis (Wuarin and Dudek, 1990; Pumford et al., 1991 and 1993; Leng et al., 1989; Brown et al., 1998). In addition, a direct effect of opioids on neuropeptide release from isolated nerve terminals has been reported by a number of studies (Summy-Long et al., 1984; Nordmann et al., 1986; Zhao et al., 1988a,b; Kato et al., 1992; Dayanithi, et al., 1992; Douglas et al., 1993). Nevertheless, the identity of the opioid receptor(s) mediating this response and the mechanism(s) used remained controversial for some time.

Opioid Inputs in the HNS

Opioid-containing axon terminals from extrinsic sources are found in the SON, PVN, and neurohypophysis (Figure 1). One possible source of endogenous opioids is the Arcuate nucleus, from which β-endorphin neurons project directly to the SON (Chronwall, 1985; Rossier et al., 1980; Leng et al., 1988a). Enkephalin-containing terminals extend to the SON from the Nucleus Tractus Solitarii, Locus Coeruleus, and ventrolateral Medulla (Russell et al., 1995). There are enkephalin-containing nerve terminals of extrinsic origin in the neurohypophysis, and this opioid is also released from the neighboring *Pars Intermedia* (Kumar et al., 1979, 1980; Rossier et al., 1980). There is also good evidence for an endogenous opioid neurotransmitter within the HNS: dynorphin $A_{(1-8)}$, the relatively κ-receptor selective opioid (Goldstein et al., 1979), is synthesized and secreted by vasopressinergic MCNs (Watson et al., 1982) and could have autocrine/paracrine feedback effects on peptide release. The same appears to be true for the relatively μ-receptor selective opioid, Met Enkephalin, which is released simultaneously with OT (Leng et al., 1994).

Methods

Isolation of Nerve Endings

Male Sprague-Dawley CD rats were sedated using CO_2 and immediately decapitated (Cazalis et al., 1987). Briefly, the animals were killed by decapitation with a guillotine following the guidelines laid down by the USA/French ethical committees and the pituitary isolated. Following removal of the anterior and intermediate lobes of the pituitary, the neural lobe was dissociated in a buffer at 37°C that contained (in mM): sucrose, 270; EGTA, 0.01; HEPES-Tris, 10, buffered at pH 7.3. The dissociated neural lobe was centrifuged at 100 x g for 1 minute, with the supernatant spun at 2400 x g for 3 minutes. The resulting pellet, containing highly purified terminals, was resuspended in Normal Locke's saline at 37°C and containing (in mM): NaCl 140; KCl 5; $CaCl_2$ 2.2; HEPES 10; Glucose 10; $MgCl_2$ 1.2; pH 7.3, and the osmolarity was 295-300 mOsmol/L. The terminals were loaded onto filters (Acrodisc, LC13, 0.45μm, Gelman Scientific, Ann Arbor, MI) where they were perfused for one hour with Locke's buffer. For the electrophysiology experiments, the centrifugation steps were omitted and the homogenate was placed directly into plastic Petri dishes. After a waiting period of 2-3 min for the terminals to settle to the bottom of the dish, the preparation was perfused with Locke's buffer to remove any floating debris.

Immunolabeling of Isolated Terminals

To identify each individual opioid receptor, the homogenate containing dissociated terminals was aliquoted equally into 35 mm polypropylene glass-bottom microwell dishes (MatTek Corporation, Ashland, MA). The tissue was fixed in 4% Paraformaldehyde-Phosphate Buffer solution (pH=7) for 30 min and washed repetitively in Phosphate buffer (PB) afterwards. To identify the presence of κ-opioid receptors, one dish was exposed to a 1%

Triton X-100 PB solution containing 10% donkey serum, an affinity purified rabbit anti-KOR at 3 μg/mL (Santa Cruz Biotechnology), an affinity purified goat anti-Neurophysin-II (AVP) at 2 μg/mL (Santa Cruz Biotechnology), and a mouse monoclonal anti-Neurophysin-I (OT) (P38) kindly provided by Dr. Harold Gainer (NIH). To identify the presence of μ-opioid receptors, another dish was exposed to a 1% Triton X-100 PB solution containing 10% donkey serum, an affinity purified rabbit anti-MOR at 3 μg/mL (Santa Cruz Biotechnology), an affinity purified goat anti-Neurophysin-II (AVP) at 2 μg/mL (Santa Cruz Biotechnology), and a mouse monoclonal anti-Neurophysin-I (OT) (P38) kindly provided by Dr. Harold Gainer (NIH). A third dish, which served as a control, was processed in identical conditions except by the omission of primary antibodies in the buffer solution. All dishes were incubated overnight, washed with PB and exposed to fluorescently-tagged secondary antibodies (Molecular Probes, Carlsbad, CA) for 3-5 hrs at room temperature. The mixture of secondary antibodies included Alexa Fluor 350 donkey anti-goat IgG, Alexa Fluor 488 donkey anti-mouse IgG and, Alexa Fluor donkey anti-rabbit IgG, 10% donkey serum in a 1% Triton X-100 PB solution. After a final series of washes the dishes were mounted with Prolong (Molecular Probes) and sealed with a glass coverslip to increase the fluorescent life of the secondary antibodies. Images were obtained with an Axiovert 200M Inverted microscope (Carl Zeiss Inc., Thornwood, New York) interfaced to a Zeiss AxioCam MRm camera fitted to a 63-X Plan/Apochromat oil immersion lens, with a numerical aperture of 1.4. Axiovert 40 (V.4.6.3.0) software was used for acquisition and image analysis. Images of one or more terminals were obtained in stacks at every 0.27 μm along the length of the terminals and deconvoluted using a high stringency fast iterative algorithm and corrected for fluorescence cross-talk between stacks. Fluorescence levels in control dishes were at or below non-specific levels for all three wavelengths (data not shown).

Peptide Release Experiments

After one hour of perfusion with Locke's saline, the terminals were perfused for another 10 min with 50 mM K^+ in the presence or absence of the drug being tested. The solutions containing elevated K^+, to stimulate active release from the terminals, were prepared by replacing an equimolar amount of NaCl with 50 mM KCl. High K^+ solution contained in (mM): NaCl 90; KCl 55; $MgCl_2$ 1.2; $CaCl_2$ 2.2; glucose 10; HEPES-Tris 10; pH 7.2; $37^{\circ}C$, and the osmolarity of the buffer was 295-300 mOsml/L. The solutions containing opioids were prepared just before they were needed. The eluate containing the released AVP and OT from the terminals was collected in 200 μl fractions and was assayed by radioimmunoassay (Cazalis et al., 1985) using specific antibodies (kindly supplied by Dr. R.J. Bicknell, Babraham Institute, Cambridge, U.K.). AVP and OT antisera were raised in sheep (the AVP antiserum was raised by Dr. Bicknell; the OT antisera by Drs. Sheldric and Flint), and the final antibody dilution was 1:100,000 for AVP and 1:25,000 for OT. The cross-reactivity of OT antiserum with AVP was 0.015%, whereas that of the AVP antiserum with OT was 0.001%. The sensitivities of the assays were 0.5 pg (AVP) and 1pg (OT). The inter- and intra-assay coefficients of variation were 5%-7% for AVP and 7%-9% for OT.

Electrophysiological Experiments

Using an inverted microscope the terminals were visually identified by their characteristic appearance, spherical shape, lack of nuclei, and relative small size (5-10 μm in diameter). For the experiments in which Ca^{2+} currents were recorded, the terminals stayed in the 2.2 mM Ca^{2+}-Locke's solution described above. For the experiments where barium currents were recorded, a solution containing $BaCl_2$ was perfused into the recording chamber right before the beginning of the recording period. This bath solution contained (in mM): $BaCl_2$ 5; NaCl 145; KCl 5; HEPES 10; Glucose 15; $MgCl_2$ 1; BSA 0.02%; pH 7.3. The terminals were patched in the perforated (Rae, et al., 1991), whole-terminal configuration (Hamill et al., 1981) using freshly prepared amphotericin B (240 μg/mL) dissolved in dimethyl sulfoxide (DMSO) and added to a pipette solution containing (in mM): Cs-glutamate 135; HEPES 10; Glucose 5; $CaCl_2$ 2; $MgCl_2$; Traethylammonium (TEA) 20; pH 7.2. In some experiments TTX ≥ 1 μM was added to the bath. Pipettes were made of thin borosilicate glass (Drummond Scientific Co., Broomall, PA) displaying resistances of 3 to 6 MΩ. Terminals were held at -80 mV and depolarized to 0 mV every 30 sec to activate the Ba-currents (I_{Ba}) using an L/M EPC-7 patch amplifier (List Electronics, Darmstadt, Germany) interfaced via TL-1 DMA Interface (Axon Instruments, Foster City, CA) to a personal computer (PC). Currents were low pass filtered at 2 kHz using an 8 pole Bessel filter (Frequency Devises Inc., Haverhill, MA) and digitized at 10 kHz. pClamp software was used for data acquisition and analysis.

Identification of Peptide Content on Isolated Individual Terminals

At the end of each electrophysiological experiment, the terminal was aspirated into the recording pipette. The pipette tip containing the terminal was broken against the bottom of a microcentrifuge tube and frozen until assayed for its neuropeptide content. Before assaying, 0.5% Triton-X 100 was added to each vial. From each vial, an aliquot was assayed for AVP and/or Oxytocin. The AVP or OT content of each terminal was determined by a specific Enzyme-Linked Immunosorbant Assay (ELISA: Assay Designs, Inc., Ann Arbor, MI). Sensitivity of the AVP and OT ELISA was 0.25 and 1 pg/well, respectively (Custer et al., 2007).

Statistical Analysis

Data are given as the mean ± s.e.m. Two-tailed student's t-tests were used to examine statistical significance of paired and unpaired data, as indicated.

Source of Chemicals

All chemicals, including DAMGO, Nicardipine and ω-conotoxin MVIIC were obtained from RBI/Sigma Chemical Co. St. Louis, MO. The ω-conotoxins GVIA and MVIIA were obtained from Molecular Probes Inc., Eugene, OR and Alomone Labs Co., Jerusalem, Israel. SNX 230 and SNX 482 were supplied by the Neurex Corporation, Menlo Park, CA. Nicardipine was first dissolved in DMSO at 0.01% of the final concentration and further diluted in Locke's buffer at 0.1 –1% before used. DAMGO and all toxins stocks were prepared in distilled water, separated in aliquots and stored at -20°C. The final working dilutions were done in Locke's buffer and used immediately, with the exception of SNX 482 that remained at room temperature for approximately 1 hr before it was used.

RESULTS

Types of Opioid Receptors in the HNS

Using autoradiography (Jordan et al., 1996), and more recently, immunolabeling techniques, two types of opioid receptors have been identified in neurohypophysial nerve terminals (Figure 2) by our group. Simultaneous exposure of isolated terminals to antibodies recognizing both types of neuropeptides as well as each opioid receptor subtype allowed us to quantify and compare the level of receptor expression between terminal types.

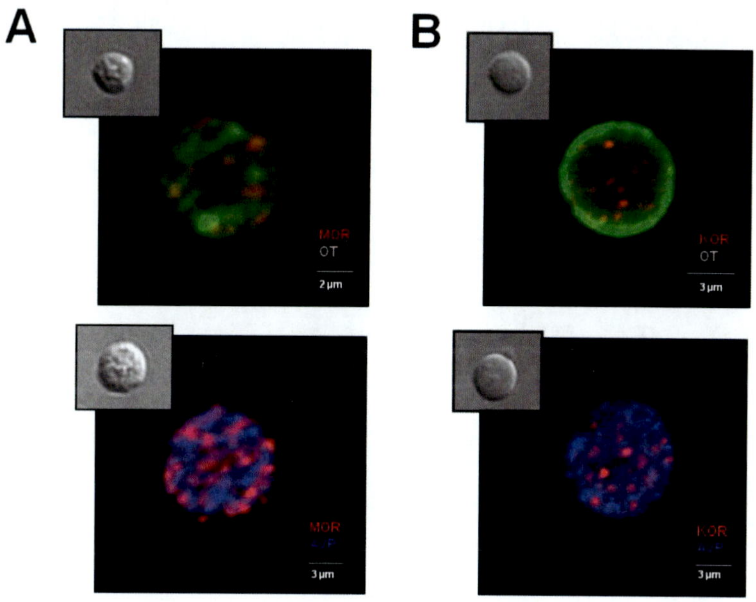

Figure 2. μ and κ opioid receptor expression in isolated NH terminals. Isolated terminals were exposed simultaneously to antibodies against neurophysin I (OT; green), neurophysin II (AVP; blue) and either an anti-κ- or anti-μ-opioid receptor (red) (see Method for a full antibody description). Bright field images of each individual terminal are shown on left, top corners. The κ-opioid receptor dependent signal intensity (SI) in OT terminals was $1.73x10^6 \pm 5.87x10^5$ gfu/μm^2 (n=22) and $9.85x10^5 \pm 4.53x10^5$ gfu/μm^2 (n=26) in AVP terminals. SI values for μ-opioid receptors were $3.02x10^6 \pm 8.85x10^5$ gfu/μm^2 (n=41) in AVP and $1.29x10^6 \pm 7.01x10^5$ gfu/μm^2 (n=50) in OT terminals. $p > 0.05$ for all groups. gfu =grey fluorescent units.

The μ-opioid receptor (MOR) dependent immunoreactivity was observed in 97.7% of AVP terminals and 99.2% of the OT terminals (n=420), while the κ-opioid receptor (KOR) dependent immunoreactivity was detected in 97.6% of AVP terminals and in 97.1% of OT terminals (n=454). Furthermore, receptor dependent signal intensities (SI) were not different between terminal types.

Opioid Effects on Presynaptic Neuropeptide Release

Opiates have been observed to decrease the secretion of both AVP and OT from the isolated, electrically stimulated neurohypophyses (Clarke et al., 1981, 1979; Hatton, 1982; Bicknell and Leng., 1981). The latter studies also provided evidence of a function for dynorphin $A_{(1-8)}$ released from AVP neurons; naloxone increased OT release from the stimulated neurohypophysis, suggesting stimuli that increase AVP (together with dynorphin) secretion *in vivo* may indirectly inhibit OT secretion (Bicknell et al., 1988). However, studies using more selective κ-opiate receptor agonists demonstrated that opiates inhibited the release of both types of neurohormones from isolated nerve endings (Nordmann et al., 1986; Zhao et al., 1988a, 1988b; Dayanithi et al., 1992).

Given the early establishment that κ-agonists were co-released with AVP *in vivo* and the belief that only this type of receptor was present in the HNS, most of the research efforts that followed were directed at describing κ-mediated effects in the HNS and thus, those actions induced by μ-opioid receptors lagged behind for some time without being addressed. More recently, our group (Ortiz-Miranda et. al., 2003, 2005) has demonstrated that depolarization-mediated neuropeptide release from NH isolated terminals in the presence of DAMGO, a selective μ-opioid receptor agonist, is inhibited in a dose-dependent manner, providing an active role for this receptor type in modulating neuropeptide release (Figure 3).

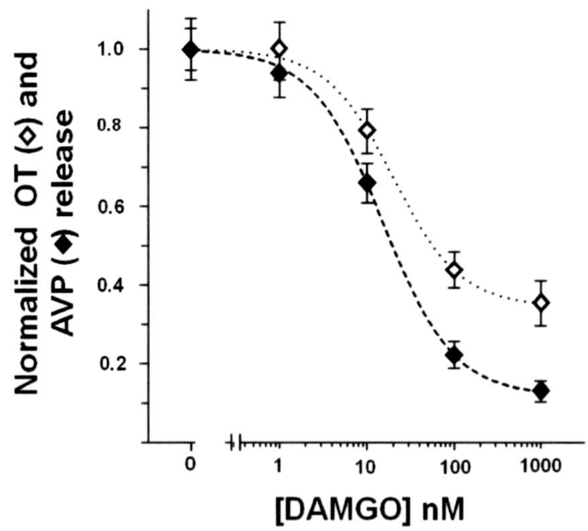

Figure 3. DAMGO can inhibit neuropeptide release in a dose-dependent manner. Isolated NH terminals were perfused with Locke's saline and exposed to increasing concentrations of DAMGO during five consecutive 50 mM high K+ stimulations. The eluate was collected in 200 mL aliquots every 5 min and immediately frozen. The amount of OT and AVP in each aliquot was determined as described in the Methods section. Mean ± s.e.m.; n=5. (Modified from Ortiz-Miranda et al., 2003).

Furthermore, when compared to AVP, oxytocin release shows a much higher sensitivity to inhibition by DAMGO. This differential sensitivity to block could imply a difference at the level of receptor expression, downstream mechanisms, or targets (*e.g.* channels) directly regulating synaptic release. Since no significant difference of the signal intensity (SI) in opioid receptor immunoreactivity was detected between terminal types, as we described in the previous section, it is most likely that receptor expression is not directly mediating the difference in sensitivity between presynaptic terminal types to DAMGO.

Calcium Channels in NH Terminals

Presynaptic voltage-gated Ca^{2+} channels are direct regulators of neurotransmitter release and a frequent target of opioids in the central and peripheral nervous systems (Macdonald and Werz, 1986; Gross and Macdonald 1987; Moises et al., 1994; Rhim and Miller, 1994; Rusin and Moises, 1995; Morikawa et al., 1995; Kanemasa et al., 1995; Knoflach et al., 1996; Hagashida et al., 1998; Adams et al., 1998; Acosta and Lopez; Su et al., 1998). In the rat neurohypophysis, four different subtypes of calcium channels comprising two major "repertoires" mediate OT *vs.* AVP release (Wang et. al., 1997, 1999). *N*- and *L*-type calcium channels seem to contribute to the release of AVP and OT equally. However, the *R*-type appears to contribute exclusively to OT release, while the *P/Q*-type mediates only AVP release (Wang et al., 1997, 1999). This channel distribution was confirmed using current measurements (Figure 4) of each component isolated by selective toxins coupled with the identification of each terminal's neuropeptide content following the recording period (see Methods section for a complete description).

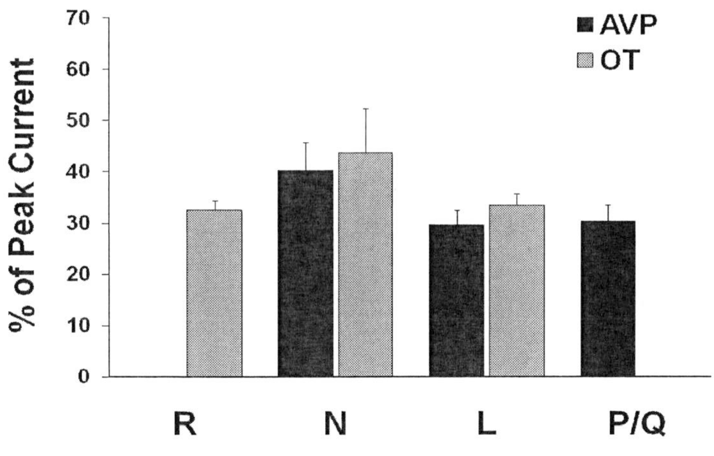

Figure 4. Distribution of Calcium channel subtypes in both types of peptidergic terminals. Percent of total peak current remaining after individual terminals were exposed to a mix of selective toxins designed to inhibit all but one calcium current type. Nicardipine (1-5μM) was used to block *L*-type channels, GVIA (500-700nM) to block *N*-type channels, SNX482 (10-25 nM) to block *R*-type channels, and SNX 230 (100-200 nM) or MVIIC (100nM) to block *P/Q* type channels. Once the currents were recorded, the terminals were suctioned inside the recording pipette and immediately frozen. Peptide content was identified using ELISAs. n = 4 to 8 per current type.

In AVP positive terminals, 30.4±3.2% of the total calcium current was contributed by *P/Q* channels, 29.7±2.8% by *L*-type channels, and 40.2±5.5% by *N*-type channels, while in OT terminals, the *R*-type channels composed 32.6±1.8%, *L*-type 33.4±2.4%, and *N*-type 43.8±8.5% of the total calcium current.

Furthermore, the use of specific calcium channel blockers to isolate individual currents was also applied to isolate the release components dependent on each individual current type. Once a particular component was isolated, we added lower and higher concentrations of DAMGO to the toxin mix to test how sensitive to μ-opioid receptor inhibition each component was.

R-Type Calcium Channels

Previous work from our laboratory demonstrated that the *R*-type channel is a highly sensitive target of the μ-opioid agonist DAMGO (Ortiz-Miranda et al., 2005). The exclusive localization of this channel type to OT-containing nerve terminals (OT+) (Figure 5A-B) provides μ-receptors with the means to inhibit OT release without having any effects on AVP release (Figure 5C-D). Calcium currents recorded from vasopressinergic (AVP+) terminals did not show an *R*-type current (Figure 5A) when all the other (*L*-, *N*-, and *Q*-type) components were selectively blocked. However, a similar mix of blockers revealed a resistant, *R*-type component in OT+ terminals which was further inhibited by 70% in the presence of low concentrations of DAMGO (Figure 5B).

In functional terms, the portion of the total OT release controlled by *R*-type channels was significantly inhibited by 10 and 100 nM DAMGO (Figure 5D), while no changes were detected in AVP release (Figure 5C), corroborating the exclusion of this calcium channel subtype in controlling its release.

DAMGO Effects on *P/Q*-Type Calcium Channels

The work of Wang et al., (1997) demonstrated that *P/Q*-type calcium channels are solely localized on AVP-containing nerve terminals and regulate exclusively the release of AVP (Figure 6). In our work, positively identified OT terminals did not express *P/Q*-type calcium currents when all other (*N*, *L*, and *R*-type) components were inhibited (Figure 6B). In AVP+ terminals, however, they composed 30% of the total current. Low concentrations of DAMGO had no effect on this current type whereas 100nM DAMGO inhibited it mildly (23%; Figure 6A). Higher concentrations of the opioid agonist were required to obtain a substantial block of this current subtype: 300 nM and 500 nM DAMGO inhibited 35% and 81% of the isolated current, respectively (data not shown), thus any targeting of this current subtype by μ-opioids will only have a relatively small functional impact in the physiological control of AVP release and most likely no effect on OT release. To corroborate this hypothesis, measurements of the *P/Q* type-dependent neuropeptide release were done in the absence and presence of DAMGO (Figure 6C-D). As expected, DAMGO did not have any significant effects on the *P/Q*-dependent OT release (Figure 6D). AVP release did not change with low (10 nM) agonist concentrations and only a small inhibitory effect on AVP release (17.6%) was detected at 100 nM DAMGO, although it remained not significantly different (p=0.2) from the toxin control values (Figure 6C). Even though higher concentrations of DAMGO were not tested in these series of experiments, the results seemed to suggest that AVP release is only modestly sensitive to 100 nM DAMGO and that much higher concentrations (>10 times higher) than those needed to block the *R*-type component are probably necessary to produce a significant inhibition.

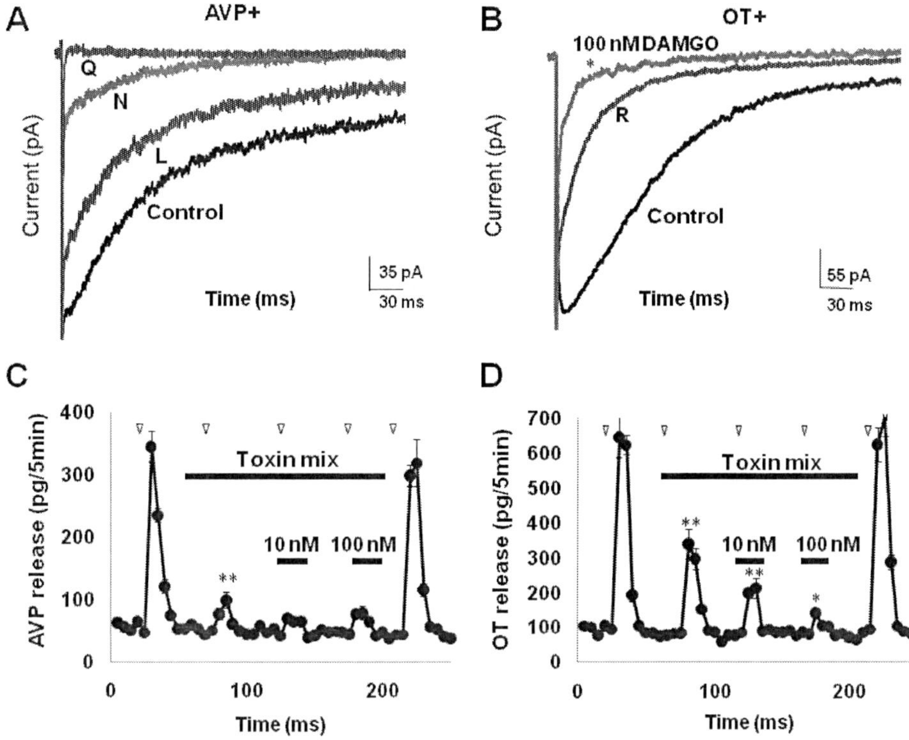

Figure 5. DAMGO can inhibit an *R*-type Ca^{2+} channel component. **A-B)** Currents were recorded from two isolated terminals in the presence of 5mM $BaCl_2$ by stepping to 10 mV from a holding potential of -80 mV using the perforated patch configuration. Once the maximum level of membrane perforation was achieved, highly specific Ca^{2+} channel toxins were applied to isolate a specific Ca^{2+} channel subtype. *L*-type, *Q*-type and *N*- type currents were blocked by 2 μM Nicardipine, 175 nM SNX230, and 500 nM GVIA, respectively. **A)** Terminal showing no resistant (*R*-type) current component and positively identified to contain AVP. **B)** Terminal showing an *R*-type current component positively identified to contain OT. In this terminal, the remaining *R*-type component was inhibited by 70% with the addition of 100 nM DAMGO. **C-D)** High K^+ stimulated neuropeptide release measured in the absence (first and last peak) and presence of DAMGO and specific Ca^{2+} channel blockers (third-fifth peaks). The toxin mix contained 2.5 μM Nicardipine, 700 nM GVIA, and 100 nM MVIIC to block *L*-type, *N*-type, and *Q*-type Ca^{2+} channels. Both OT and AVP were measured from identical aliquots. Open triangles denote high K^+ stimulations. **C)** An 84 ± 6.3% reduction on AVP release was obtained by the toxin treatment. Further stimulation in the presence of 10 nM or 100 nM DAMGO did not caused any significant decrease in AVP release (p=0.1 and p=0.9, respectively). A complete recovery is shown in the last release peak after both toxins and DAMGO are washed away. **D)** OT release was decreased 52.5 ± 3.7% by the toxin treatment and further exposure to 10 nM and 100 nM DAMGO caused a 57.3% and 79.5% reduction in *R*-type dependent OT release, respectively. A complete recovery to the initial control values is shown in the last release peak. n=3; mean ± s.e.m. *=p<0.05; **p<0.01. (Modified from Ortiz-Miranda et al., 2005).

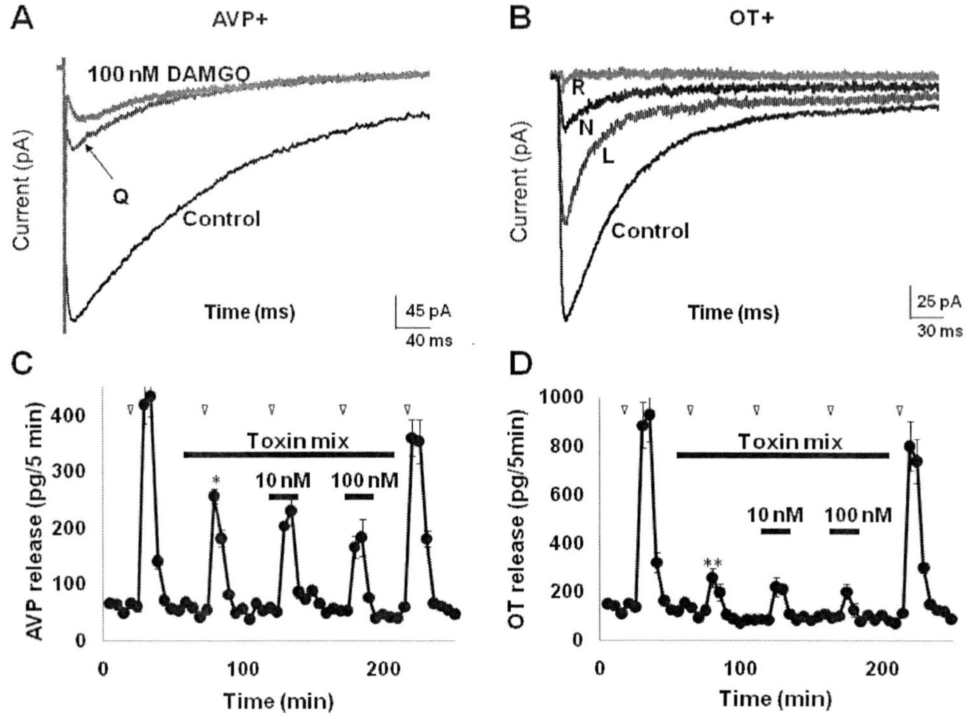

Figure 6. *P/Q*-type channels are modestly inhibited by DAMGO. **A-B**) The *P/Q*-type Ca^{2+} channels were isolated pharmacologically by selectively blocking all other components as described previously. Currents were recorded as described in Figure 5 using 500 nM GVIA, 2 μM Nicardipine, and 25 nM SNX482 to block *N*-type, *L*-type and *R*- type currents respectively. **A**) In this AVP+ terminal, 100 nM DAMGO blocks 32% of the isolated *P/Q*-type current component. Similar percentages (30.4 ± 3.2%) were obtained in other four AVP identified terminals. **B**) Current records from an OT+ terminal showing no residual *P/Q* type component after all other current types were blocked. **C-D**) High K^+ stimulated neuropeptide release mediated by *P/Q* type channels was measure in the presence of 2.5 μM Nicardipine, 700 nM GVIA, and 10 nM SNX482 (second through fourth peaks) and 10 and 100 nm DAMGO (third and fourth peaks, respectively). First and last peaks are controlled stimulations without any drug present. Both peptides are measured from identical aliquots. Open triangles denote high K^+ stimulations. **C**) AVP release was significantly reduced to 53.2 ± 4.6% on by the toxin treatment. Exposure to 10 nM DAMGO did not cause any significant change in the *P/Q*-type dependent AVP release but further stimulation with 100 nM DAMGO caused a small (17.6 ± 9.6%) decrease in AVP release. An almost complete recovery to initial control values is shown in the last release peak after both toxins and DAMGO are washed away. **D**) OT release declined to 73.2 ± 7.1% in the presence of the *L*-, *N*-, and *R*-type blockers. The small residual component was not sensitive to either 10 ($p=0.9$) or 100 nM DAMGO ($p=0.1$) (third and fourth peaks). A full recovery of OT release was obtained after all toxins and DAMGO are washed away. n=4; mean ± s.e.m. *$p<0.05$, **$p<0.01$.

DAMGO Effects on *L*-Type Calcium Channels

Isolated *L*-type currents, present in both AVP-containing (Figure 7A) and OT-containing (Figure 7B) terminals proved to be also minimally sensitive to DAMGO. Both types of neuropeptide-containing terminals displayed an *L*-type component ranging between 30-33% of the total calcium current using either the pharmacological approach (with toxins) described previously or a depolarized membrane potential (-40 mV) to isolate this component (Lemos and Nowycky, 1987; Wang et al., 1992). Vasopressin-containing terminals were particularly insensitive to 100 nM DAMGO, and as a general rule, we found that much higher concentrations of DAMGO were needed (≥ 200 nM) to produce a detectable (≥ 6%) inhibitory effect.

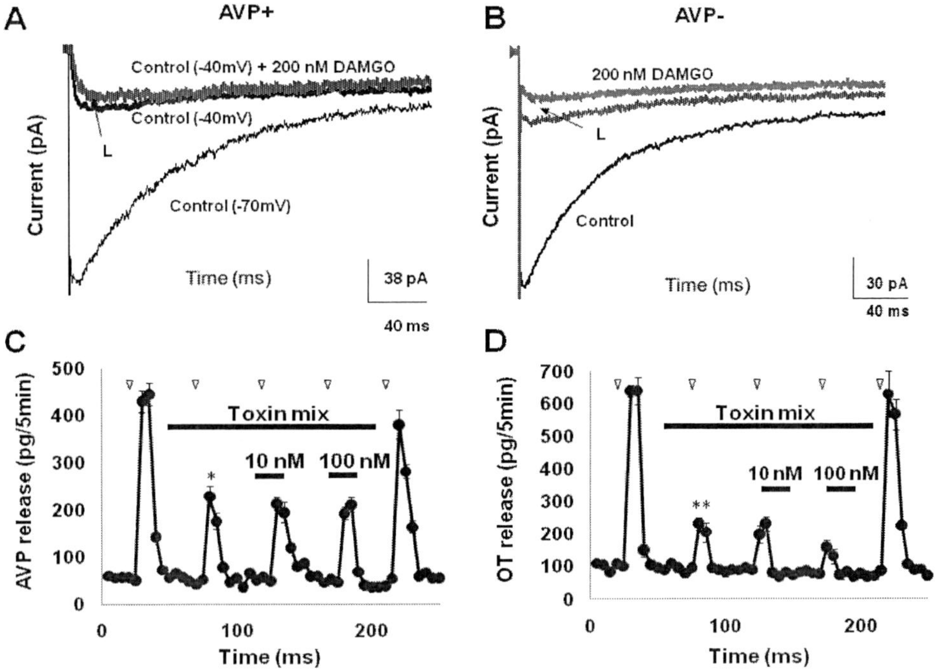

Figure 7. *L*-type calcium channels are minimally affected by DAMGO. **A-B)** *L*-type Ca^{2+} channel currents were recorded from isolated terminals in the presence of 5 mM $BaCl_2$ using two distinct methods to isolate this current. Step pulses to +10mV were applied for 300ms in both cases. **A)** Terminal held at –40mV to inactivate all other Calcium currents and isolate the *L*-type current component. The control trace shows the total amount of current at –70mV. Exposure to 200 nM DAMGO blocks <10% of the voltage-isolated *L*-type current. Similar results (6 ± 12.7%) were obtained in five AVP+ terminals. **B)** *L*-type currents were isolated using 500 nM GVIA, 175 nM SNX230, and 25 nM SNX482 to block the *N*-type, *Q*-type and *R*- type currents, respectively. Further exposure to 200 nM DAMGO caused a 20.7% reduction of this current component. This AVP- terminal was assumed to contain OT since it was negative for the presence of AVP (see Custer et al., 2007). Similar values (15 ± 4.8%) were obtained in three more OT identified terminals. **C-D)** High K^+ elicited neuropeptide release measured in the absence and presence of 700 nM GVIA, 100 nM MVIIC, and 10 nM SNX230 to block *N*-type, *Q*-type, and *R*-type Ca^{2+} channels (second through fourth peaks) and DAMGO (third and fourth peaks). First and fifth peaks are used as control stimulations. Both neuropeptides were measured from the same experimental samples. Open triangles denote high K^+ stimulations. **C)** AVP release was significantly reduced by 54.1 ± 2.3% with the toxin treatment. Exposure to 10 nM DAMGO did not cause any significant inhibition of the *L*-type dependent AVP release however, 100 nM DAMGO caused a small 9.4% reduction of this release component. An almost complete recovery is shown in the last high K^+ stimulation after both toxins and DAMGO are washed away. **D)** OT release was significantly reduced to 23.8±2.3% by the toxin mix and 10 nM DAMGO did not cause any further changes. At 100 nM DAMGO the inhibition of this isolated component reached 12.2±1.9%. A complete recovery is shown in the last control stimulation. n=4; mean ± s.e.m. *$p<0.05$, **$p<0.01$.

On the other hand, OT-containing terminals were slightly more sensitive to the μ-opioid agonist, with 100 nM DAMGO inducing a 15.2 ± 4.8% decrease, 200 nM a 20.7% decrease, and 300 nM a 32% decrease of the *L*-type isolated component (not shown).

The effects of DAMGO on the *L*-type dependent neuropeptide release were fairly similar to those observed on isolated *L*-type calcium currents (Figure 7C-D). Since voltage cannot be used to isolate this component during the release measurements, toxin blockers were used exclusively in these experiments. The vasopressin release component was significantly decreased to ~54% of control values in the presence of the *N*-, *Q*-, and *R*-type calcium channel blockers. At low concentrations of DAMGO, no further inhibition beyond the initial isolated component level was visible, while at 100 nM only a marginal 9.4 ± 3.6% inhibition of the *L*-type dependent AVP release was obtained (Figure 7C). The OT release component was only slightly more sensitive to DAMGO than AVP (Figure 7D) in these experiments. Beyond the 76% reduction in OT release obtained by the toxin mix, no further effects were observed at 10 nM DAMGO and only a 12% inhibition was detected with 100 nM DAMGO. Thus, μ-opioid targeting of this channel subtype is very modest and is evidently not differentially attained between OT and AVP terminals.

DAMGO Effects on *N*-Type Calcium Channels

A very distinctive behavior was observed in isolated *N*-type calcium currents exposed to DAMGO (Ortiz-Miranda et al., 2010). Each peptidergic terminal type showed a prominent disparity in current sensitivity to low (~10nM) *vs*. high (~100nM) concentrations of the μ-opioid agonist (Figure 8). AVP+ terminals exposed to low concentrations of DAMGO exhibited a 30-66% current increment of the isolated N-type component (Figure 8A), while the higher opioid concentration induced either small current increases or non-significant decreases. In general, the bell-shaped responses of this current component to DAMGO peaked (at least in the conditions used for the electrophysiological recordings) at concentrations close to 100 nM DAMGO. Increasing concentrations of the agonist induced smaller current enhancements and eventually led to inhibition (Ortiz-Miranda et al., 2010). On the other hand, the isolated *N*-type current component in OT+ terminals was always inhibited by DAMGO (Figure 8B). Low agonist concentrations reduced the isolated *N*-type currents by 7% whereas 100 nM DAMGO blocked 29% of the current. Thus, the divergence in the responses to μ-opioid agonists suggests that both types of neuropeptides could be differentially affected by the physiological activation of this receptor.

As would be predicted by the current measurements, the *N*-type dependent release component proved to be significantly different for each type of neuropeptide (Figure 8C-D). Low concentrations of DAMGO enhanced the *N*-type dependent AVP release by 27.9%, while higher concentrations of the agonist became inhibitory (Figure 8C). As we anticipated, OT was decreased by 64.4% and 77.6% in the presence of 10 nM and 100 nM DAMGO, respectively (Figure 8D). Thus, μ-opioid targeting of the *N*-type channel subtype could mediate and/or fine-tune distinct responses in physiological conditions where only the release of one neuropeptide is needed.

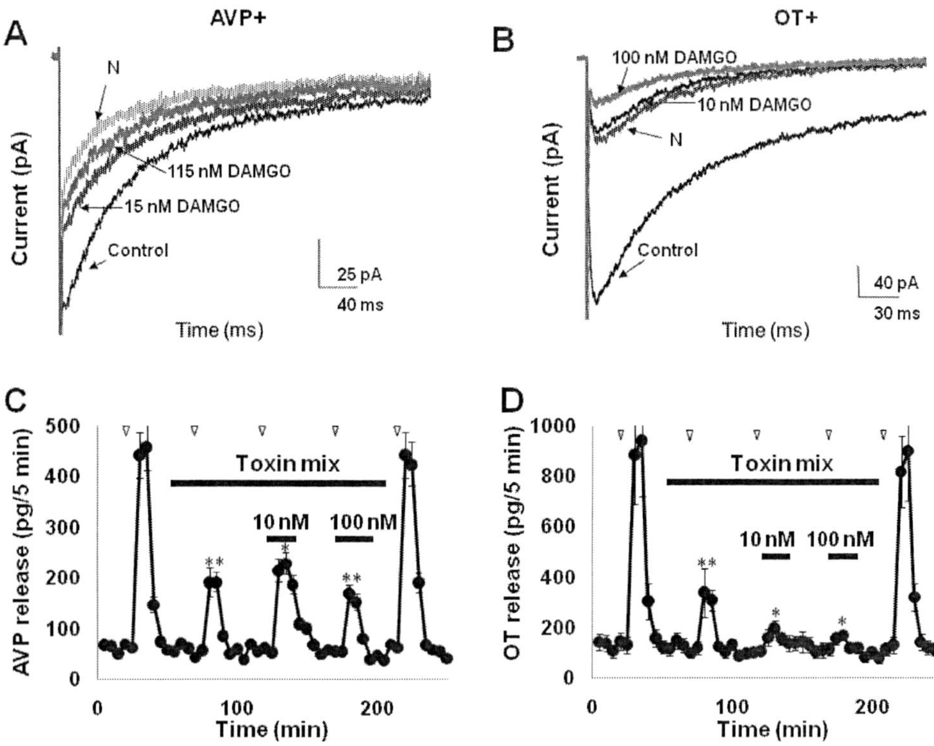

Figure 8. DAMGO effects on isolated *N*-type currents vary with terminal's peptide identity. **A-B**) *N*-type mediated currents were recorded from isolated terminals in the presence of 5mM $BaCl_2$ using identical stimulation protocols and isolated pharmacologically by selectively blocking all other current components as previously described. *P/Q*-type, *L*-type and *R*- type currents were blocked by 175 nM SNX230, 2 μM Nicardipine, and 25 nM SNX482 respectively. **A**) An AVP+ terminal expressing 40% *N*-type isolated currents. Low, 15 nM DAMGO enhanced the isolated currents by 30%, while a higher 115 nM concentration caused a smaller 16% increment of the isolated N-type component. **B**) An OT+ terminal expressing 37.7% N-type isolated current. This component was inhibited by 6.8% at 10 nM DAMGO and by 28.9% at 100 nM DAMGO. **C-D**) High K^+ elicited neuropeptide release measured in the absence and presence of DAMGO and specific Ca^{2+} channel blockers. Notice that both neuropeptides were measured from the same experimental samples. Open triangles denote high K^+ stimulations. **C**) AVP release was measured in the absence (first peak) and presence of 2 μM Nicardipine, 100 nM MVIIC, and 10 nM SNX482 to block *L*-type, *Q*-type, and *R*-type Ca^{2+} channels (second though fourth peaks). A significant reduction of 51.2 ± 2.9% on AVP release was obtained with the toxin treatment. Exposure to 10 nM DAMGO caused a significant 27.9% increase and 100 nM DAMGO a significant 45% reduction in AVP release. Last stimulation shows an almost complete recovery of the release responses. **D**) In the presence of the toxin mix, OT release was significantly reduced by 64.8%. Exposure to 10 nM and 100 nM DAMGO caused a 59% and 64% reduction of OT release, respectively. Post control stimulation shows full recovery of the responses. Mean ± s.e.m; n=3 to 4; ** $p<0.01$ and * $p<0.05$. (Modified from Ortiz-Miranda et al., 2010).

DISCUSSION

Given the typical mixed anatomical distribution of cell bodies and nerve endings containing OT and AVP in the HNS (Ben-Barak et al., 1985; Mezey and Kiss, 1991), it is expected and unavoidable that endogenous opiates either co-released with neuropeptides or locally released by other afferent nerves will most likely reach both AVP and OT terminals concurrently. Thus, a mechanism that discriminates or fine tunes differential presynaptic responses for each neuropeptide is an essential characteristic of the system to ensure proper physiological responses.

Targeting channels in direct control of regulating synaptic release, such as calcium channels, is thus a very efficient way to achieve this objective. Even though we do not fully know what downstream messenger systems may control μ-opioid receptor signaling to each channel subtype in the HNS at this point, we can provide a general mechanism that describes how differential responses to DAMGO can be attained in each type of nerve ending. A summary of all the changes induced by 10 and 100 nM DAMGO on all calcium channel subtypes and their underlying release components is shown in Figure 9.

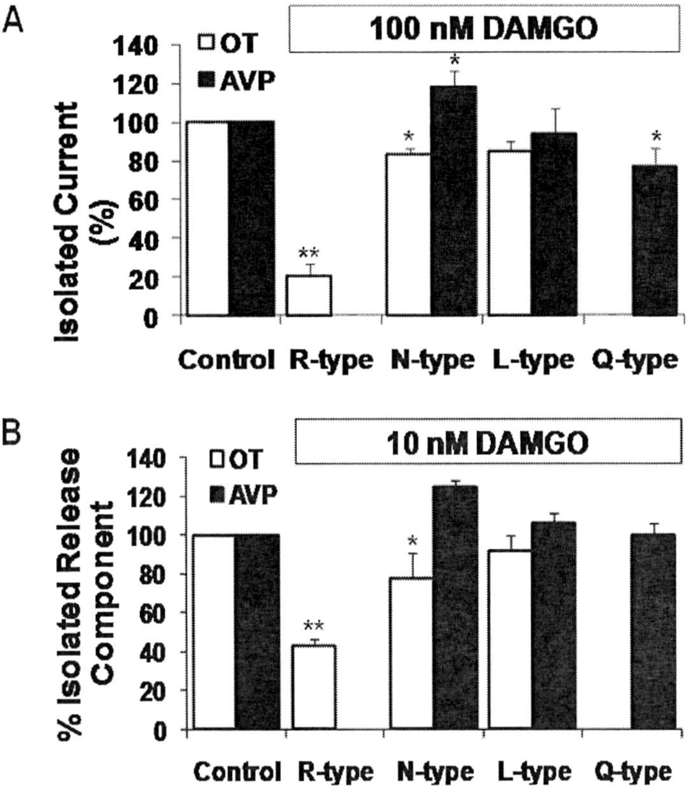

Figure 9. Summary of DAMGO's induced changes on calcium currents and neuropeptide release in isolated terminals. **A**) DAMGO's effect on Ca^{2+} channels in identified MCN terminals. All currents were normalized to the isolated current value and only terminals identified (OT+, AVP+ or AVP-) were included in this summary. In OT identified terminals 100 nM DAMGO inhibited 78.7 ± 8.1% (n=3); of *R*-type calcium channels; 27 ± 3% (n=3) of the *N*-type calcium channels; and, 15 ± 4.8% (n=4) of *L*-type channels. This same concentration of DAMGO induced 23.3 ± 8.8% (n=4) inhibition of *Q*-type calcium channels; 66.7± 8.3% (n=6) increase of the *N*-type calcium channels; and, 6.2 ± 12.7% (n=5) of *L*-type channels in AVP+ terminals. **B**) Summary of DAMGO's effect on AVP/OT release in MCN terminals. All amounts were normalized to the release level obtained for each isolated component before any opioid was applied. At 10 nM DAMGO, OT-dependent release on *R*-type, *N*-type and *L*-type calcium channels were inhibited by 57%, 29%, and 8%, respectively. The AVP-dependent release on *Q*-type and *L*-type was not significantly affected. However, the *N*-type dependent AVP release was increased by 30% at this agonist concentration. Mean ± s.e.m.

Each bar in the histogram depicting the effects of 100 nM DAMGO on calcium currents was normalized to the isolated current values. In terminals positively identified to contain OT, 100 nM DAMGO blocked 79% of the *R*-type, 27% of the *N*-type and 15% of *L*-type calcium channels (Figure 9A).

Similar inhibition values (57%, 29%, and 8%) were observed on each isolated OT release component, respectively, by DAMGO (Figure 9B). Thus, only net inhibitory effects on OT containing terminals are produced by DAMGO. On the other hand, in AVP-containing terminals, *P/Q*-type channels were blocked by 23% and *L*-type channels by <10%, but the *N*-type current increased up to 66%; a pattern of behavior that was recapitulated in the release measurements with enhancements of the *N*-type component and small changes in the *P/Q*- and *L*- type components. Therefore, the net effect of DAMGO on AVP release would depend on the summation of all the inhibitory and stimulatory responses of those channels controlling its release and the relative concentration of μ-opioid agonists present.

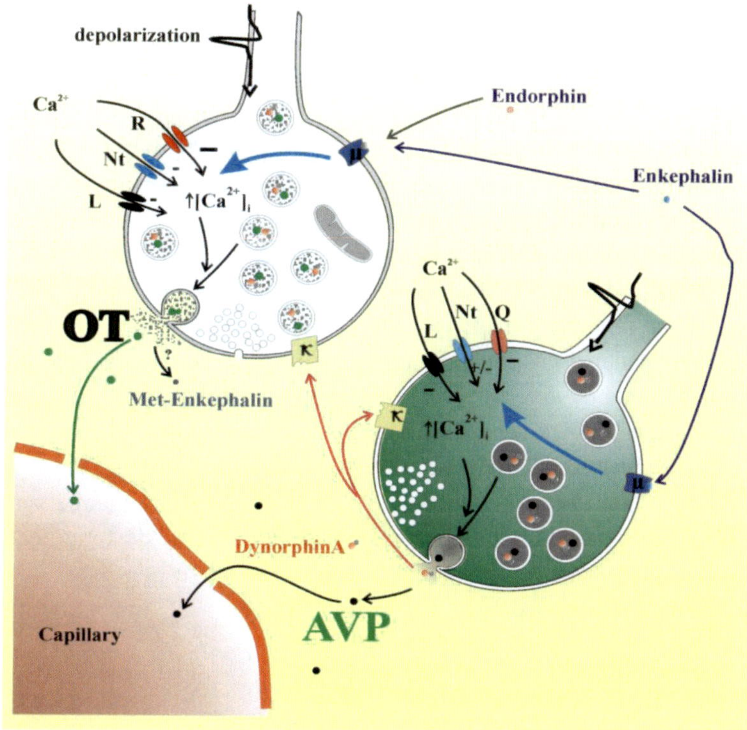

Figure 10. **Proposed model for** μ-opioid receptor activation on OT and AVP releasing Magnocellular nerve endings. Locally released agonists activate opioid receptors in both OT and AVP containing terminals, by a yet unknown mechanism, able to regulate the influx of calcium during a depolarizing stimulus. The net calcium influx is determined by the sum of all types of voltage-gated Ca^{2+} channel mediating the stimulated release of each neuropeptide. Oxytocin's **higher sensitivity** to DAMGO comes as a result of the general inhibition of all channels (*R*-, *N*-, and *L*-type) controlling its release. In an analogous way, the reduced sensitivity of AVP containing terminals to DAMGO, particularly at low concentrations of the agonist, could also be explained by a limited block of *L*-, and *P/Q*-type channels, coupled to an unusual potentiation of the *N*-type calcium current.

Based on these results, we propose a simple model in Figure 10 that illustrates the main conclusions attained on the μ-opioid modulation of AVP *vs.* OT release in the neurohypophysis. We propose that the relative sensitivity to μ-opioid inhibition of OT release, particularly at lower agonist concentrations, is due to a net inhibitory action on all voltage-gated channels mediating calcium influx in an OT terminal.

In contrast, an AVP terminal will respond with little or no change in release to lower concentrations of the μ-opioid agonist, as some of the voltage-gated channels controlling calcium influx are inhibited and others are potentiated. At higher concentrations of the agonist, those channels controlling AVP release that were not affected before or were potentiated become increasingly inhibited; thus, a net inhibition of calcium influx can be obtained. This simple model by itself is able to explain the shift in μ-opioid dependent inhibition observed in the response curves for AVP and OT release (Ortiz-Miranda et. al., 2003).

The next obvious question to answer, and one with a potentially interesting response, pertains to the kind of signaling cascade that μ-opioid receptors use to produce simultaneous enhancements and inhibitions on very closely localized channels within a membrane area. Preliminary evidence indicates that high concentrations of μ-opioid agonists induce inhibition of peptide release by a mechanism that is voltage-independent (Velazquez-Marrero et al., 2010) and involves a second messenger cascade leading to rises in $[Ca^{2+}]i$ in NH terminals (Ortiz-Miranda et al., 2010). The presence of $G\alpha_{q/11}$ in NH terminals (Velazquez-Marrero et al., 2008), provides a potential candidate to test as a mediator of these inhibitory effects. Finally, the role of kinases and/or other activators of soluble intracellular second messenger pathways are currently being explored as targets of μ-opioid activation. In AVP+ terminals, we envision a mechanism that activates a distinct cellular pathway, available only to AVP+ terminals at low μ-opioid agonist concentrations, that is overpowered at higher concentrations by the activation of an inhibitory pathway such as the ones postulated above (Ortiz-Miranda et al., 2010). In this scenario, *N*-type calcium channels play an interesting, key role in their versatility to be modulated by diverse G protein dependent pathways.

In conclusion, we have shown how opioid effects on voltage-gated calcium channels can directly mediate differences in the control of neurohypophysial OT and AVP release. These mechanisms and pathways used by each type of terminal to control channel activity, $[Ca^{2+}]_{i,}$ and thus the net amount of neuropeptide released from these presynaptic endings not only help us understand the physiology of the HNS and how it responds to opiates, but also represent potential strategies used by other neurons in the CNS to regulate their synaptic output.

Acknowledgments

Supported by NIH grants DA10487 to JRL and UMass FDSP Grant P60037094900000 to SOM.

References

Acosta CG, Lopez HS (1999) δ-Opioid receptor modulation of several voltage-dependent Ca2+ currents in rat sensory neurons. *J. Neurosci.* 19:8337-8348.

Adams DJ, Trequattrini C (1998) Opioid receptor-mediated inhibition of ω-conotoxin GVIA-sensitive calcium currents in rat intracardiac neurons. *J. Neurophysiol.* 79:753-762.

Acher R & Chauvet J (2002) Organismal handling of water balance in vertebrates. *Symp. Soc. Exp. Biol.* 54:169-182.

Baylis PH (1987) Osmoregulation and control of vasopressin secretion in healthy humans. *Am. J. Physiol.* 253:R671-678.

Ben-Barak Y, Russell JT, Whitnall MH, Ozato K, Gainer H (1985) Neurophysin in the hypothalamo-neurohypophysial system. 1. Production and characterization of monoclonal antibodies. *J. Neurosci.* 5:81–97.

Bicknell RJ, Leng G, Russell JA, Dyer RG, Mansfield S, Zhoa B (1980) Hypothalamic opioid mechanisms controlling oxytocin neurones during parturition. *Brain Res. Bull.* 20:743-749.

Bicknell RJ, Leng G (1981) Relative efficiency of neural firing patterns for vasopressin release in vitro. *Neuroendocrinology* 33:295-299.

Bicknell RJ, Leng G, Lincoln DW, Russell JA (1988) Naloxone excites oxytocin neurones in the supraoptic nucleus of lactating rats after chronic morphine treatment. *J. Physiol.* 396:297-317.

Brown CH, Ludwig M, Leng G (1998) Kappa-opioid regulation of neuronal activity in the rat supraoptic nucleus in vivo. *J. Neurosci.* 18:9480-9488.

Cazalis, M., Dayanithi, G., and Nordmann, J.J (1985) The role of pattern burst and interburst interval on the excitation-coupling mechanism in the isolated rat neural lobe. *J. Physiol.* (London) 369: 45-60.

Cazalis M, Dayanithi G, Nordmann JJ (1987) Hormone release from isolated nerve endings of the rat neurohypophysis. *J. Physiol.* (Lond) 390:55-70.

Chrobak JJ, Napier TC (1993) Opioid and GABA modulation of accumbens-evoked ventral pallidal activity. *J. Neural. Transm.* 93: 123-143.

Chronwall, BM (1985) Anatomy and physiology of the neuroendocrine arcuate nucleus. *Peptides* 6:1-11.

Clarke G, Wood P, Merrick L, Lincoln DW (1979) Opiate inhibition of peptide release from the neurohumoral terminals of hypothalamic neurones. *Nature* 282:746-748.

Clarke G, Noble R, Wakerley JB (1981) Effects of morphine on the discharge of supraoptic neurones recorded from rat hypothalamic slices in vitro. *J. Physiol.* 319:115P-116P.

Custer EE, Ortiz-Miranda S, Knott TK, Rawson R, Elvey C, Lee RH, Lemos JR (2007) Identification of the neuropeptide content of individual rat neurohypophysial terminals. *J. Neurosci. Methods* 163(2): 226-34.

Dayanithi G, Stuenkel EL, Nordmann JJ (1992) Intracellular calcium and hormone release from nerve endings of the neurohypophysis in the presence of opioid agonists and antagonists. *Exp. Brain Res.* 90:539-545.

DeBodo RC (1944) The antidiuretic action of morphine, and its mechanism. *J. Pharmcol. Exp. Ther.* 82:74-85.

Douglas AJ, Dye S, Leng G, Russell JA (1993) Endogenous opioid regulation of oxytocin secretion through pregnancy in the rat. *J. Neuroendocrinol.* 5:307-314.

Goldstein A, Tachibana S, Lowney LI, Hunkapiller M and Hood L (1979) Dynorphin (1 13), an extraordinarily potent opioid peptide. *Proc. Natl. Acad. Sci. USA* 76:6666-6670.

Gross RA, Macdonald RL (1987) Dynorphin A selectively reduces a large transient (N-type) calcium current of mouse dorsal root ganglion neurons in cell culture. *Proc. Natl. Acad. Sci. USA* 84:5469-5473.

Hagashida H, Hoshi N, Knijnik R, Zadina JE, Kastin AJ (1998) Endomorphins inhibit high-threshold Ca2+ channel in rodent NG108-15 cells overexpressing μ-opioid receptors. *J. Physiol.* (Lond) 507:71-75.

Hamill OP, Marty A, Neher E, Sakmann B, Sigworth SJ (1981) Improved patch-clamp techniques for high resolution current recording from cells and cell-free membrane patches. *Pflügers. Arch.* 391:85-100.

Hartman RD, Rosella-Dampman LM, Emmert SE, Summy-Long JY (1986) Ontogeny of opioid inhibition of vasopressin and oxytocin release in response to osmotic stimulation. *Endocrinology* 119:1-11.

Hartman RD, Rosella-Dampman LM, Summy-Long JY (1987) Endogenous opioid peptides inhibit oxytocin release in the lactating rat after dehydration and urethane. *Endocrinology* 121:536-543.

Hatton, GI (1982) Phasic bursting activity of rat paraventricular neurons in the absence of synaptic transmission. *J. Physiol.* 327:273-284.

Hughes J, Smith TW, Kosterlitz HW, Fothergill L, Morgan BA, Morris HR (1975) Identification of two related pentapeptides from the brain with potent opiate agonist activity. *Nature* 258: 577-579.

Jordan D, Tafani JA, Ries C, Zajac JM, Simonnet G, Martin D, Kopp N, Allard M (1996) Evidence for multiple opioid receptors in the human posterior pituitary. *J. Neuroendocrino*l. 8: 883-887.

Kanemasa T, Asakura K, Ninomiya M (1995) Kappa-opioid agonist U50488 inhibits P-type Ca2+ channels by two mechanisms. *Brain Res.* 702:207-212.

Kato M, Chapman C, Bicknell RJ (1992) Activation of κ-opioid receptors inhibits depolarization-evoked exocytosis but not the rise in intracellular calcium in secretory nerve terminals of the neurohypophysis. *Brain Res.* 574:138-146.

Knoflach F, Reinscheid RK, Civelli O, Kemp JA (1996) Modulation of voltage-gated calcium channels by orphanin FQ in freshly dissociated hypocampal neurons. *J. Neurosci.* 16:6657-6664.

Koob GF (1992) Drugs of abuse: anatomy, pharmacology and function of reward pathways. *Trends Pharmacol. Sci.* 13: 177-184.

Kumar MSA, Chen, CL and Muther, TF (1979) Changes in the pituitary and hypothalamic content of methionine enkephalin during the estrus cycle of the rat. *Life Sci.* 25:1687-1696.

Kumar MSA, Chen CL and Huang HH (1980) Pituitary and hypothalamic concentration of metenkephalin in young and old rats. *Neurobiol. Aging* 1:153-155.

Lemos JR, Nowycky MC (1989) Two types of calcium channels coexist in peptide releasing vertebrate nerve terminals. *Neuron* 2:1419–26.

Lemos JR (2001) Magnocellular Neurons. In: *Nature Encyclopedia of Life Sciences*. London: Nature Publishing, http://www.els.net/ [doi:10.1038/ npg.els.0000176]: A176, 1-5.

Leng G, Mansfield S, Bicknell RJ, Dean ADP, Ingram CD, Marsh MIC, Yates JO, Dyer RG (1985) Central opioids: a possible role in parturition. *J. Endocrinol.* 106:219-224.

Leng G, Mansfield S, Bicknell RJ, Brown D, Chapman C, Hollingsworth S, Ingram CD, Marsh MIC, Yates JO, Dyer RG (1987) Stress-induced disruption of parturition in the rat may be mediated by endogenous opioids. *J. Endocrinol.* 114:247-252.

Leng G, Yamashita H, Dyball REJ, Bunting R (1988a) Electrophysiological evidence for a projection from the arcuate nucleus to the supraoptic nucleus. *Neurosci. Lett.* 89:146-151.

Leng G, Mansfield S, Bicknell RJ, Blackburn RE, Brown D, Chapman C, Dyer RG, Hollingsworth S, Shibuki K, Yates JO, Way S (1988b) Endogenous opioid actions and effects of environ-mental disturbance on parturition and oxytocin secretion in rats. *J. Reprod. Fert.* 84:345-356.

Leng G, Russell JA, Grossman R (1989) Sensitivity of magnocellular oxytocin neurones to opioid antagonist in rats treated chronically with intracerebroventricular (icv) morphine. *Brain Res.* 484:290-296.

Leng G, Bicknell RJ, Brown D, Bowden C, Chapman C and Russell JA (1994) Stimulus induced depletion of pro enkephalins, oxytocin and vasopressin and pro enkephalin interaction with posterior pituitary hormone release in vitro. *Neuroendocrinology* 60:559-566.

Leng G, Brown CH, Russell JA (1999) Physiological pathways regulating the activity of magnocellular neurosecretory cells. *Prog. Neurobiol.* 57:625-655.

Lewis ME, Khachaturian H, Watson SJH (1985) Combined autoradiographic-immunocytochemical analysis of opioid receptors and opioid peptide neuronal systems in brain. *Peptides* 6: 37-47.

Lohmeier T (2003) Neurohypophysial hormones. *Am. J. Physiol. Regul. Integr. Physiol.* 285:R715-R717.

Macdonald RL, Werz MA (1986) Dynorphin A decreases voltage-dependent calcium conductance of mouse dorsal root ganglion neurons. *J. Physiol.* 377:237-249.

Mansour A, Khachaturian H, Lewis ME, Akil H, Watson SJ (1989) Anatomy of CNS opioid receptors. *Trends Neurosci.* 11: 308-314.

Mansour A, Fox CA, Akil H, Watson SJ. (1995) Opioid-receptor mRNA expression in the rat CNS: anatomical and functional implications. *Trends Neurosci.* 18: 22-29.

Mezey E, Kiss JZ (1991) Coexpression of vasopressin and oxytocin in hypothalamic supraoptic neurons of lactating rats. *Endocrinology* 129(4):1814–20.

Moises HC, Rusin KI, Macdonald RL (1994) μ- and κ-opioid receptors selectively reduce the same transient components of high-threshold calcium current in rat dorsal root ganglion sensory neurons. *J. Neurosci.* 14:5903-5916.

Morikawa H, Fukuda K, Kato S, Mori K, Higashida H (1995) Coupling of the cloned μ-opioid receptor with the ω-conotoxin-sensitive Ca2+ current in NG108-15 cells. *J. Neurochem.* 65:1403-1406.

Nordmann JJ, Dayanithi G, Cazalis M (1986) Do opioid peptides modulate, at the level of the nerve endings, the release of neurohypophysial hormones? *Exp. Brain Res.* 61:560-566.

Oiso Y, Iwasaki Y, Kondo K, Takatsuki K, Tomita A (1988) Effect of the Opioid □kappa-receptor agonist U50 488H on the secretion of arginine vasopressin. Study on the mechanism of U50 488H-induced diuresis. *Neuroendocrinology* 48:658-662.

Ortiz-Miranda SI, Dayanithi G, Coccia VJ, Custer E, Alphandery S, Mazuc E, Treistman SN, Lemos JR (2003) μ-opioid receptor modulates peptide release from rat neurohypophysial terminals by inhibiting Ca2+ influx. *J. Neuroendocrinol.,* 15:888-894.

Ortiz-Miranda SI, Dayanithi G, Custer E, Treistman SN, Lemos JR (2005) μ-opioid receptor preferentially inhibits oxytocin release from neurohypophysial terminals by blocking R-type Ca2+ channels. *J. Neuroendocrinol.,* 17:583-90.

Ortiz-Miranda S, Dayanithi G, Velazquez-Marrero C, Treistman SN, and Lemos JR (2010). Differential modulation of N-type calcium channels by μ-opioid receptors in oxytocinergic vs. vasopressinergic neurohypophysial terminals. *J. Cell Physiol.*: 225: 276–288.

Paronis CA, Ko M, Sobczyk-Kojiro K, Mosberg HI, Woods JH (1995) Effects of norbinaltorphimine (nBNI) and quartenary anologs of nBNI on CI-977-induced diuresis and analgesia. *Soc. Neurosci. Abs.* 21:1362.

Pert, CB Pasternak, GW and Snyder, SH (1973) Opiate agonists and antagonists discriminated by receptor binding in brain. *Science* 182:1359-1361.

Pumford KM, Leng G, Russell JA (1991) Morphine actions on supraoptic oxytocin neurones in anaesthetized rats: tolerance after i.c.v. morphine. *J. Physiol.* (Lond) 440:437-454.

Pumford KM, Russell JA, Leng G (1993) Effects of the selective kappa-opioid agonist U50, 488 upon the electrical activity of supraoptic neurones in morphine-tolerant and morphine-naïve rats. *Exp. Brain Res.* 94:237-246.

Rae J, Cooper K, Gates P, Watsky M (1991) Low access resistance perforated patch recordings using amphotericin B. *J. Neurosci. Meth.* 37: 15-26.

Rhim H, Miller RJ (1994) Opioid receptors modulate diverse types of calcium channels in the nucleus tractus solitarius of the rat. *J. Neurosci.* 14:7608-7615.

Rossier J, Pittman Q, Bloom F and Guillemin R (1980) Distribution of opioid peptides in the pituitary: a new hypothalamic pars nervosa enkephalinergic system. *Fed. Proc.* 39:2555-2560.

Rusin KI, Moises HC (1995) μ-Opioid receptor activation reduces multiple components of high-threshold calcium current in rat sensory neurons. *J. Neurosci.* 15:4315-4327.

Russell JA, Gosden RG, Humphreys EM, Cutting R, Fitzsimons N, Johnston S, Liddle S, Scott S, Stirland JA (1989) Interruption of parturition in rats by morphine: a result of inhibition of oxytocin secretion. *J. Endocrinol.* 121:521-536.

Russell JA, Leng G, Bicknell RJ (1995) Opioid tolerance and dependence in the magnocellular oxytocin system: a physiological mechanism? *Exp. Physiol.* 80: 307-340.

Russell JA, Leng G, Douglas AJ (2003) The magnocellular oxytocin system, the fount of maternity: adaptations in pregnancy. *Frontiers Neuroendocrinol.* 24:27-61.

Schoffelmeer AN, Mulder AH (1994) Functional studies on opioid receptor heterogeneity in the central nervous system. *Neurochem. Int.* 24: 433-437.

Self DW, Nestler, EJ (1995) Molecular mechanisms of drug reinforcement and addiction. *Annu. Rev. Neurosci.* 18:463-495.

Su X, Wachtel RE, Gebhart GF (1998) Inhibition of rat colon sensory neurons by κ- but not μ- or δ-opioids. *J. Neurophysiol.* 80:3112-3119.

Summy-Long JY, Miller DS, Rosella-Dampman LM, Hartman RD, Emmert SE (1984) A functional role for opioid peptides in the differential secretion of vasopressin and oxytocin. *Brain Res.* 309(2):362-366.

Velázquez-Marrero C, Ortiz-Miranda S, Marrero HG, Lemos JR (2008) μ-Opioid signaling via ryanodine-sensitive Ca2+ stores in isolated terminals of the Neurohypophysis. *Soc. for Neurosci. Abst.* 865.29.

Wang G, Thorn P, Lemos JR (1992) A novel large-conductance Ca2+-activated potassium channel and current in nerve terminals of the rat neurohypophysis. *J. Physiol.* 457:47–74.

Wang G, Dayanithi G, Kim S, Hom D, Nadasdi L, Kristipati R, Ramachandran J, Stuenkel, EL, Nordmann JJ, Newcomb R, Lemos JR (1997) Role of Q-type Ca2+ channels in vasopressin secretion from neurohypophysial terminals of the rat. *J. Physiol.* 502:351-33.

Wang G, Dayanithi G, Newcomb R, Lemos JR (1999) An R-type Ca2+ current in neurohypophysial terminals preferentially regulates oxytocin secretion. *J. Neurosci.* 19:9235-9241.

Watson SJ, Akil H, Fischli W, Goldstein A, Zimmerman E, Nilaver G and vanWimersm Greidanus TB (1982) Dynorphin and vasopressin: common localization in magnocellular neurons. *Science* 216:85-87.

Wuarin J-P, Dudek FE (1990) Direct effects of an opioid peptide selective for μ-receptors: intracellular recordings in the paraventricular and supraoptic nuclei of the guinea-pig. *Neuroscience* 36:291-298.

Zamponi GW, Bourinet E, Nelson D, Nargeot J, Snutch TP (1997) Crosstalk between G proteins and protein kinase C mediated by the calcium channel alpha1 subunit. *Nature* 385(6615): 442-446.

Zhao BG, Chapman C, Bicknell RJ (1988a) Opioid-noradrenergic interactions in the neurohypophysis I. Differential opioid receptor regulation of oxytocin, vasopressin, and noradrenaline release. *Neuroendocrinol.* 48:16-24.

Zhao BG, Chapman C, Bicknell RJ (1988b) Functional κ-opioid receptors on oxytocin and vasopressin nerve terminals isolated from the rat neurohypophysis. *Brain Res.* 462:62-66.

In: Opioids: Pharmacology, Clinical Uses and Adverse Effects ISBN 978-1-61942-101-1
Editors: Djavakhi Tvildiani and Kakha Gegechkori

Chapter 4

SYNERGY ABILITIES OF SPINAL OPIOIDS RECEPTORS: A NOVEL APPROACH FOR POLYANALGESIC THERAPY?

Itsaso Buesa and Jon Jatsu Azkue
Department of Neurosciences, School of Medicine and Dentistry, The University of the Basque Country, Barrio Sarriena s/n, 48940 Leioa, Spain

ABSTRACT

Reduced clinical efficacy of opioid analgesic drugs in chronic pain, including neuropathic pain, remains an unsolved issue. Since the spinal dorsal horn is a major site of opioid pain modulation, new insights into molecular opioid mechanisms may provide novel avenues for chronic therapy.

The reported experimental evidence supports the view that the efficacy of opioid ligands to depress nociceptive neurotransmission in dorsal horn neurons may be modified as a result of interaction with other receptors in the same family as well as with other receptor families. In this chapter we review conditions for potential interactions in a variety of experimental models.

Available data from two experimental models of pathological pain, namely the long-term potentiation of spinal C fiber-evoked potentials and surgical ligature of the fifth spinal nerve, support that spinal hyperexcitation may activate an endogenous factor that can enhance the effectiveness of spinally acting opioid ligands. Further, the spinal mu or delta opioid receptors undergo profound functional changes as a result of peripheral nerve injury, which are largely yet not exclusively attributable to tonic co-activation of the mu opioid receptor. Potentially involved mechanisms based on receptor-interactions as well as possible implications are discussed.

INTRODUCTION

Increased sensitivity to painful stimuli (hyperalgesia) and painful sensation to innocuous stimuli (allodynia), which are common symptoms in neuropathic pain, are thought to be attributable, at least in part, to impairment of spinal inhibitory systems acting postsynaptically or impinging upon primary afferent fiber to spinal second order neurone synapses (Millan, 1999; Woolf and Salter, 2000; Zimmermann, 2001).

The spinal dorsal horn is critically involved in pain transmission and is a major site for opioid analgesic effect (Dickenson, 1995; Chen and Pan, 2006). Here, endogenous opioids act through at least three distinct G-protein-coupled opioid receptors (GPCR) subtypes termed μ opioid receptor (MOR), δ opioid receptor (DOR), and κ opioid receptor (KOR). Almost all GPCR agonists that have an analgesic action are coupled to Gi/o proteins (Pan et al., 2008). Activation of MOR and DOR profoundly inhibits glutamate release from the primary afferent terminals to spinal dorsal horn neurons (Kohno et al., 1999) and both MOR and DOR agonists produce dose-dependent inhibition of C fiber-evoked firing activity of spinal dorsal horn neurons in response to noxious stimuli (Dickenson et al., 1987; Sullivan et al., 1989). In addition to opioid receptors, a variety of other GPCRs can modulate inhibitory neurotransmission at the spinal level, including NPY receptors (Y1, Y2), cannabinoid receptors (CB1, CB2), adenosine- (A1), acetylcholine- (AChR), serotonin- (5-HT) and γ-aminobutyric acid$_B$ (GABA$_B$) receptors, as well as metabotropic glutamate receptors and noradrenergic receptors (Pan et al., 2008; Taylor, 2009).

It is now recognized that GPCRs can form oligomeric complexes in addition to the traditionally envisaged monomeric species (Taylor, 2009). Many GPCRs are capable of forming different dimer combinations to interact with G-proteins, thereby affecting diverse intracellular signaling pathways and various ion channels (Pan et al., 2008). These associations can result in novel pharmacological properties distinct from either component receptor, including enhancement of ligand binding affinity, changes in functional coupling and altered receptor trafficking (George et al., 2002; Bulenger et al., 2005). Understanding the molecular mechanisms involved in synergistic interactions of these receptors is of both clinical and theoretical importance to devise more efficacious therapies for pain management.

Synergistic Interaction between Spinal MOR and DOR during Sustained Pain

Although the mechanisms whereby nerve injury results in loss of opioid efficacy remain to be established, increased spinal excitability and intrinsic changes in spinal cord opioid mechanisms are likely to play a role (Dickenson and Suzuki, 2005). We have shown that higher concentrations of spinally applied morphine are required to suppress field potentials evoked in the spinal dorsal horn by noxious afferent input in states of spinal hyperexcitability such as the spinal nerve ligation (SNL) model of neuropathic pain and long-term potentiation (LTP) of C fiber-evoked spinal field potentials (Buesa et al., 2008a,c). Spinal transmission of C fiber-input can be diminished by classical opioid morphine after induction of LTP of synaptic strength between primary C afferent neurones and spinal second order neurones by electrically elicited peripheral nerve input, either intravenously administered (Tanabe et al., 2006) or spinally applied at higher doses (Buesa et al., 2008c). This is suggestive that abnormal pain involving some forms of synaptic plasticity in the spinal cord, including perceptual correlates of LTP, may be responsive to morphine with sufficient dose escalation (Dickenson and Suzuki, 2005). However, the rate of depression of spinal responses by spinally administered opioids may not be linearly correlated with the level of spinal excitation. For example, ongoing spinal LTP appears to activate an endogenous factor leading to an enhancement of morphine depression only when spinal field potential areas elicited by C fiber-input largely exceed the pre-conditioning baseline (Buesa et al., 2008c). Analogously, we have shown that the potency of the DOR- but not MOR or KOR agonists is strikingly increased following SNL, relative to sham-operated animals (Buesa et al., 2008a). Further, pharmacological MOR stimulation facilitates spinal DOR-activity, strongly suggesting that DOR facilitation after SNL may be due to endogenous activation of the spinal MOR (Buesa et al., 2008a).

The spinal DOR may be antihyperalgesic in neuropathic pain. Although DOR density is decreased in laminae I-II following ligation of spinal L5/6 nerves (Stevens et al., 1991; Stone et al., 2004), intrathecally delivered (D-Ala2)-Deltorphin II suppresses thermal hyperalgesia and effectively attenuates mechanical allodynia in the chronic constriction injury model (Mika et al., 2001; Holdridge and Cahill, 2007). Consistently, DOR deficient mice undergo severe thermal and mechanical allodynia after sciatic nerve ligation (Nadal et al., 2006), suggesting that the modulatory role of spinal DOR may be crucial in neuropathic pain. Notably, DOR-mediated antinociception may be greater in neuropathic than in control rats (Holdridge and Cahill, 2007).

Can Descending Pathways Enhance the Depressing Effect of MOR and DOR?

Central delivery of nociceptive information is critically dependent on interaction of peripheral input reaching spinal second order neurones with both segmentally and suprasegmentally organized modulatory circuits, the latter including axon projections to the spinal cord that largely arise from the brainstem (Basbaum and Fields, 1978; Zhuo and Gebhart, 1991; Yoshimura and Furue, 2006).

One candidate mechanism involved therein may be a synergistic interaction of exogenously administered morphine with descending inhibitory pathways activated by high spinal excitation, e.g. hyperexcitation induced by conditioning HFS (Buesa et al., 2008c). Electrical, high intensity conditioning stimulation preferentially activates descending inhibitory, rather than facilitatory controls (Porreca et al., 2002; Suzuki et al., 2002). This suggests that the reported clinical inefficacy of morphine in states of enhanced spinal excitation, including neuropathic pain, may not be due to a decrease in morphine inhibition rates, but rather related to the higher background excitation level to overcome (Buesa et al., 2008c). Consistent with this view, spinal MOR blockade disinhibited C fiber-evoked spinal field potentials in SNL rats, but not in non-ligated ones, supporting that SNL model and sustained pain triggers endogenous MOR ligand release by descending inhibitory systems (Levine et al., 1977; Kayser and Guilbaud, 1990; Buesa et al., 2008a). This is also consistent with the observed mechanical allodynia following intrathecal CTOP delivery in neuropathic rats (Back et al., 2006) but not in uninjured ones (Keck et al., 1995; Mizoguchi et al., 1995). Interestingly, DOR regulation may not depend on endogenous ligand release (Gendron et al., 2007), and we have previously reported that spinal superfusion with the DOR antagonist naltrindole fails to disinhibit C fiber-evoked field potentials in SNL rats and therefore that nerve injury is not capable of triggering tonic activation of the spinal DOR (Buesa et al., 2008a).

A mechanism potentially involved in enhancing the depressing effect of DOR on spinal nociception may be formation of opioid receptor dimers in neurons (Salahpour et al., 2000), including heterodimers (Jordan and Devi, 1999; George et al., 2000). Dimer formation can alter ligand-binding properties and functional effects (Jordan and Devi, 1999; Charles et al., 2003). Tonic activation of MOR/DOR complexes in the spinal cord can tonically inhibit high voltage-gated Ca^{+2} channels mediated by Gi/o proteins (Pan et al., 2008). Regarding this potential mechanism, it is known that DOR and MOR are co-localized in dorsal root ganglia as well as in perikarya and primary afferents terminals in superficial dorsal horn laminae (Egan and North, 1981; Arvidsson et al., 1995). In the spinal cord, enkephalins potentiate MOR antinociception (Malmberg and Yaksh, 1992), presumably by activating a DOR/MOR complex (Traynor and Elliot, 1993), as the two subtypes are thought to form receptor heterodimers in which DOR ligand binding is facilitated by MOR activation (Gomes et al., 2000). The ability of MOR to modulate DOR activity (Gendron et al., 2007) may account for the positive interaction between the two receptors in depressing spinal nociception that can be induced in the absence of nerve injury by simultaneous activation by appropriate agonist drugs (Buesa et al., 2008a). The spinal MOR becomes tonically active following SNL, probably by endogenous ligand, which may at least partly account for the increased ability of DOR to depress peripherally evoked dorsal horn field potentials after SNL (Buesa et al., 2008a).

Formation of MOR/DOR Heterodimers Requires Interaction with G-proteins

The concept of dimerization of GPCRs is well established (Gurevich and Gurevich, 2008; Milligan, 2004). However, the role of this molecular mechanism on activation and regulation of effector systems is still unclear. GPCRs do not necessarily exist in the same state of oligomerization from biosynthesis to degradation. Indeed, they may exist as monomers, homodimers, or heterodimers in the Golgi apparatus, on the cell surface membrane, and/or in the process of internalization (Gurevich and Gurevich, 2008). Dimerization may occur after receptor activation on the surface membrane, and this process may influence surface expression in neurons that express both MOR and DOR. For example, heterodimerization is a prerequisite for translocation of the $GABA_B$ receptor and other GPCRs from the endoplasmic reticulum to the Golgi apparatus or to the cell membrane (Margeta-Mitrovic et al., 2000; Terrillon et al., 2003; Hague et al., 2004). Therefore, the possibility of G-proteins being involved in the interactions between MOR and DOR deserves attention. Activation of one of the receptors forming a heteromeric complex may influence conformational stability of the other in the active state, thereby modulating efficacy of G-protein activation. Therefore, G-proteins might play a role not only in determining ligand selectivities but also in mediating synergistic effects on downstream signaling (Gomes et al., 2000).

DOR are mainly localized to the cytoplasm, in what has been suggested to constitute a *reserve pool* of receptors that may be inserted into the plasma membrane in response to physiological changes (Zhang et al., 1998; Cahill et al., 2001a,b; Bao et al., 2003; Cahill et al., 2003). Activation of DOR by agonist-binding has been shown to trigger a slow but long-lasting exocytosis of large dense core vesicles (Wang et al., 2008), leading to an increase in cell surface area and most likely coupling with other OR receptors. Golgi chaperone protein

RTP4 and/or other chaperone proteins or receptor activity-modifying proteins (RAMPs) could participate in a heterodimer-specific component of MOR biosynthesis and transport to the DRG surface membrane (Bulenger et al., 2005; Walwyn et al., 2009).

Interaction of MOR and DOR with G-proteins appears to be a critical step in heterodimer formation (Law et al., 2005). There is substantial evidence suggesting that MOR and DOR can couple to a variety of G-proteins (George et al., 2000; Gomes et al., 2000, 2004; Fan et al., 2005; Law et al., 2005). For instance, opioids can act through various G-proteins to activate phospholipase C (PLC), thereby mobilizing Ca^{+2}, activating PKC and enhancing presynaptic voltage-gated, ATP-gated and Ca^{+2}- and K^{+} channel activity (for review see Aantaa et al., 1995; Connor and Christie, 1999; Millan, 1999, 2002; Law et al., 2000). There are two secretory pathways in neurons, namely the regulated and the constitutive pathways (De Camilli and Jahn, 1990; Jung and Scheller, 1991). Recent studies have shown that most DORs in dorsal root ganglion neurons are localized to the cytoplasm (Evans et al., 1992; Kieffer et al., 1992) and insertion of DORs into the plasma membrane may be associated with regulation of exocytosis by membrane depolarization (Huang and Neher, 1996; Bao et al., 2003). In addition, DOR agonist-induced receptor externalization via PLC could be involved in modulation of morphine tolerance. Stimulation of DOR expression on DRG neuron surfaces is associated with reduced morphine tolerance (Guan et al., 2005). It is noteworthy that the human DOR F27C polymorphism, which reduces receptor maturation efficiency and cell surface expression, is associated with higher risk of substance dependence and acute thermal pain sensitivity (Kim et al., 2004; Zhang et al., 2008; Leskelä et al., 2009). Additional studies are required to determine whether this polymorphism disrupts MOR/DOR dimerization and hinders MOR receptor biosynthesis (Walwyn et al., 2009).

Opioid Receptors Are Prone to Association with Other Neurotransmitter Receptors

The ability of the DOR agonist (D-Ala2)-Deltorphin II to depress dorsal horn responses to noxious input increases dramatically after SNL, an increase that is only partially reproduced in intact rats by co-administration of the MOR antagonist CTOP (Buesa et al., 2008a). These findings are important in that they anticipate the involvement of additional, as yet unidentified endogenous factors that contribute to enhancing DOR-mediated analgesia during sustained pain. Although further studies are needed to clarify this, potential candidates may include cannabinoid- (Reche et al., 1996; Welch and Stevens, 1992), serotoninergic-, muscarinic-, α2 adrenergic- (Kovelowski et al., 1999) purinergic receptors (Cahill et al., 1996) and $GABA_B$ receptor (Buesa et al., 2008b), some of which will be addressed in the following sections. An additional implication for this is that, if antinociception by exogenously administered opioid drugs proves to at least partly be dependent on a positive interaction with descending pain inhibitory systems, then a novel candidate pathogenic pathway contributing to poor response to opioids may be an impaired function of descending inhibition, which has been mechanistically implicated in a variety of idiopathic clinical pain syndromes (Edwards, 2005).

Morphine-Induced Depression of Spinal Excitation is not Altered Following Acute Disruption of $GABA_B$ Receptor Activity

GABA is a major inhibitory neurotransmitter that is widely distributed throughout the central nervous system. GABA activates 3 pharmacologically distinct types of receptors, namely ionotropic $GABA_A$ and $GABA_C$ receptors and G-protein-coupled $GABA_B$ receptors (Bowery, 1993; Bowery and Enna, 2000). Based on neuroanatomical data, excitation elicited in dorsal horn neurones by C fiber-input may be modulated concurrently at the level of neurotransmitter release both by GABA and opioid receptors, as central processes of unmyelinated fibers contain the μ opioid receptor (Ji et al., 1995) and also are a likely localization of the $GABA_B$ receptor (Malcangio and Bowery, 1993; Marvizon et al., 1999).

We found spinal superfusion with morphine to effectively depress field potentials mediated by C fibers during spinal disinhibition induced by $GABA_B$ antagonist CGP35348, with IC50 values for MOR not differing from naïve rats (Buesa et al., 2008b). Furthermore, no interaction was found to occur between CGP35348 and MOR treatments as independent variables (Buesa et al., 2008b). This was suggestive that MOR efficacy may not be altered by $GABA_B$ receptor blockade, and consistent with the observation that effective MOR doses may be primarily dependent on the level of previous excitation (Saeki and Yaksh, 1993). At the clinical level, this would imply that adequate analgesia may be achieved even with increased spinal cord excitability with sufficient dose escalation (Dickenson and Suzuki, 2005). These findings did not support decreased spinal inhibition mediated by $GABA_B$ receptor as an underlying pathogenic mechanism accounting for reduced opioid analgesia in neuropathic pain.

Synergistic Interaction between Opioid - and Adrenergic Receptors

Receptors of the α2 type (α2AR) can be classified into three distinct but highly homologous, subtypes, namely $\alpha2_A$, $\alpha2_B$, and $\alpha2_C$, all of which are coupled to pertussis-toxin-sensitive Gi/o proteins (Bylund et al., 1994 and for reviews see Aantaa et al., 1995; MacDonald et al., 1997; Philipp et al., 2002). Synergistic interactions have been well documented for DOR/$\alpha2_A$AR (Stone et al., 1997; Grabow et al., 1999; Alguacil and Morales, 2004), MOR/$\alpha2_A$AR (Roerig et al., 1992; Stone et al., 1997), and DOR/$\alpha2_C$AR (Fairbanks et al., 2002; Guo et al., 2003). Although molecular mechanisms involved in these synergistic interactions are still unclear, it has been shown that DOR and the $\alpha2_A$AR are co-expressed on the axon terminals of primary afferent fibers in the spinal dorsal horn and that protein kinase C mediates a synergistic interaction between the two receptors in vivo (Overland et al., 2009). Co-expression of these receptors provide an anatomical substrate for analgesic synergy, perhaps due to protein-protein interactions such as hetero-oligomerization (Riedl et al., 2009).

Interactions between Cannabinoid and Opioid Receptors

Cannabinoid receptors CB1 and CB2 are present at key sites involved in the relay and modulation of nociceptive information in the central nervous system, and analgesic effects of cannabinoids have been well documented. CB1 receptors are densely expressed in the superficial dorsal horn of spinal cord (Tsou et al., 1998; Salio et al., 2002). CB1 and CB2 receptors mediate anti-hyperalgesic and anti-nociceptive effects in a variety of inflammatory, post-operative or neuropathic pain states (Kelly et al., 2003; Elmes et al., 2004; Sagar et al., 2005; Taylor, 2009). Both receptors are coupled to the Gi/o family of G-proteins and both inhibit adenylyl cyclase in most tissues and cells (Howlett et al., 1986).

Inactive doses of delta 9-tetrahydrocannabinol, a cannabinoid CB1 receptor agonist, have been demonstrated to enhance the potency of opioids such as morphine (Cichewicz et al., 1999; Cichewicz, 2004). Although potentiation of morphine analgesia by delta 9-tetrahydrocannabinol may be due to release of endogenous opioid peptides (Corchero et al., 1997), an interaction at the intracellular signal transduction level has also been proposed since cannabinoid and opioid receptors both are coupled to the same G-proteins (De Vries et al., 1991; Rubino et al., 2000; Shapira et al., 2000; Salio et al., 2001). By using double immunocytochemical labeling, it has been shown that some spinal interneurons co-express CB1 and MOR (Salio et al., 2001), and that both of them can form heterodimers in heterologous expression systems (Hojo et al., 2008; Rizzo et al., 2004). Although the DOR may also be involved in opioid/cannabinoid interactions (Welch and Stevens, 1992; Reche et al., 1996), their mutual regulation in nociceptive transmission is not clear.

Spinal Muscarinic - and Opioid Receptor Interactions

Molecular cloning studies have revealed 5 distinct muscarinic acetylcholine receptors (mAChR) referred to as M1-5 (Caufield, 1993; Wess et al., 2003). These receptors are linked to Gi/o proteins (Caulfield, 1993; Fields and Casey, 1997; Wess et al., 2003). M2, M3 and M4, but not M1 subtypes are present in the superficial dorsal horn (Duttaroy et al., 2002; Li et al., 2002). Activation of mAChR inhibits the response of spinal dorsal horn projection neurons to nociceptive stimuli in rats (Chen and Pan, 2004).

Receptor-binding studies suggest that the functional activity of spinal M4 receptor is dependent on the presence of the M2 subtype, possibly indicating the existence of functional M2/M4 mAChR oligomers in the spinal cod (Chen et al., 2005). The mAChRs also mediates some of the antinociceptive effects of opioids (Chen and Pan, 2001) and can enhance the analgesic effect of systemic opioids in humans (Hood et al., 1997). Interestingly, it has been reported that spinal muscarinic receptor subtypes M2 and M4 contribute to morphine antinociception during thermal stimulation in mice (Honda et al., 2004).

Synergistic Interaction between OR and Serotonin Receptors

Seven families of 5-HT receptors (5-HT1 through 5-HT7) have so far been identified (for a review, see Nichols and Nichols, 2008). Some of these, including 1–4, and 7, are contained in spinal dorsal horn neurones (Marlier et al., 1991; Kidd et al., 1993; Hoyer et al., 1994; Wu et al., 2001; Wang et al., 2003; Doly et al., 2005). Except for the ionotropic 5-HT3 receptor, all 5-HT receptors are G-protein-coupled receptors that can modulate ligand- and voltage-gated channels (Nichols and Nichols, 2008).

The 5-HT1 receptor class leads to neuronal hyperpolarization by inhibiting adenyl cyclase via activation Gi/o protein and subsequent augmentation and reduction, respectively, of K^+ channel and Ca^{+2} channel permeabilities (Nichols and Nichols, 2008). Influence of the receptor on antinociception may be dual. On the one hand, the presence of subtypes 5-HT1A (Wu et al., 2001; Wang et al., 2003) and 5-HT1B (Wu et al., 2001) in primary afferent neurones may be expected to inhibit neurotransmitter release and thus to reduce nociception, whereas on the other, 5-HT1A receptor- expression in spinal GABAergic and enkephalinergic neurones (Wu et al., 2001; Wang et al., 2003) may be seen as anticipating disinhibition of nociception.

Results from our laboratory provide evidence for a dramatic increase in analgesic potency of 5-HT1A agonist after SNL (Aira et al., 2010). One way of interpreting this change may be in connection with an autoreceptor role of serotonin class 1 receptors (Matsumoto et al., 1992; Nichols and Nichols, 2008). We observed disinhibition of C fiber-evoked potentials by spinal application of 5-HT1A receptor-antagonist (S)-WAY 100135 in SNL, but not in sham operated rats, which is indicative that 5-HT1A may become tonically active during sustained pain (Aira et al., 2010). Like for most other GPCRs, there is now evidence that serotonin receptors can form dimers in both cell culture and endogenous systems (Nichols and Nichols, 2008). Western blot experiments have demonstrated that 5-HT1B and 5-HT1D receptors, which share a high degree of homology, each form homodimers when expressed separately but form heterodimers when heterologously expressed in the same cell (Xie et al, 1999). It is not unconceivable that activation of descending inhibitory pathways may promote formation of heterodimeric complexes consisting of MOR, DOR, and 5-HT receptors of subtypes 1B or 1A in spinal dorsal horn neurons.

Conclusion

Exploitation of drug synergies is important in clinical pain management, since administration of lower drug doses may help reduce unwanted side effects. Available evidence supports the occurrence of functional synergies between neurotransmitter receptors in spinal cord neurons. Heterodimerization properties of opioid receptors confer this family an extremely complex pharmacology, which is difficult to understand as a mere result of isolated genetic products. Opioid receptor heterodimerization, especially with other spinal GPCRs provides a versatile mechanism whereby the cell generates a new *target-receptor* with specific properties distinct from those of their monomers/homodimers. On these grounds, the precise identification and functional characterization of OR homo- and heterodimers in the central nervous system constitutes a promising goal that could open new avenues for the treatment of neurophatic and persistent pain.

Acknowledgments

Supported by the Government of the Basque Country under program SAIOTEK (SA-2010/00110) and by Ayudas a Grupos de Investigación del Sistema Universitario Vasco.

References

Aantaa, R; Marjamäki, A; Scheinin, M. Molecular pharmacology of alpha 2-adrenoceptor subtypes. *Ann. Med.*, 1995 27, 439-449.

Aira, Z; Buesa, I; Salgueiro, M; Bilbao, J; Aguilera, L; Zimmermann, M; Azkue, JJ. Subtype-specific changes in 5-HT receptor-mediated modulation of C fibre-evoked spinal field potentials are triggered by peripheral nerve injury. *Neuroscience*, 2010 168, 831-841.

Alguacil, LF; Morales, L. Alpha-2 adrenoceptor ligands and opioid drugs: pharmacological interactions of therapeutic interest. *Current Neuropharmacology,* 2004 2, 343-352.

Arvidsson, U; Dado, RJ; Riedl, M; Lee, JH; Law, PY; Loh, HH; Elde, R; Wessendorf, MW. Delta-Opioid receptor immunoreactivity: distribution in brainstem and spinal cord, and relationship to biogenic amines and enkephalin. *J. Neurosci.*, 1995 15, 1215-1235.

Back, SK; Lee, J; Hong, SK; Na, HS. Loss of spinal mu-opioid receptor is associated with mechanical allodynia in a rat model of peripheral neuropathy. *Pain,* 2006 123, 117–126.

Bao, L; Jin, SX; Zhang, C; Wang, LH; Xu, ZZ; Zhang, FX; Wang, LC; Ning, FS; Cai, HJ; Guan, JS; Xiao, HS; Xu, ZQ; He, C; Hökfelt, T; Zhou, Z; Zhang, X. Activation of delta opioid receptors induces receptor insertion and neuropeptide secretion. Neuron, 2003 37, 121-133.

Basbaum, AI; Fields, HL. Endogenous pain control mechanisms: review and hypothesis. *Ann. Neurol.*, 1978 4, 451-162.

Bowery, NG; Enna, SJ. gamma-aminobutyric acid(B) receptors: first of the functional metabotropic heterodimers. *J. Pharmacol. Exp. Ther.*, 2000 292, 2-7.

Bowery, NG. GABAB receptor pharmacology. *Annu. Rev. Pharmacol. Toxicol.*, 1993 33, 109-447.

Buesa, I; Urrutia, A; Aira, Z; Salgueiro, M; Bilbao, J; Mozas, M; Aguilera, L; Zimmermann, M; Azkue, JJ. Depression of C fibre-evoked spinal field potentials by the spinal delta opioid receptor is enhanced in the spinal nerve ligation model of neuropathic pain: involvement of the mu-subtype. *Neuropharmacology*, 2008a 55, 1376-1382.

Buesa, I; Urrutia, A; Bilbao, J; Aguilera, L; Zimmermann, M; Azkue, JJ. Morphine-induced depression of spinal excitation is not altered following acute disruption of GABA(A) or GABA(B) receptor activity. *Eur. J. Pain*, 2008b 12, 677-685.

Buesa, I; Urrutia, A; Bilbao, J; Aguilera, L; Zimmermann, M; Azkue, JJ. Non-linear morphine-induced depression of spinal excitation following long-term potentiation of C fibre-evoked spinal field potentials. *Eur. J. Pain*, 2008c 12, 814-817.

Bulenger, S; Marullo, S; Bouvier, M. Emerging role of homo- and heterodimerization in G-protein-coupled receptor biosynthesis and maturation. *Trends Pharmacol. Sci.*, 2005 26, 131-137.

Bylund, DB; Eikenberg, DC; Hieble, JP; Langer, SZ; Lefkowitz, RJ; Minneman, KP; Molinoff, PB; Ruffolo, RR Jr; Trendelenburg, U. International Union of Pharmacology nomenclature of adrenoceptors. *Pharmacol. Rev.*, 1994 46, 121-136.

Cahill, CM; McClellan, KA; Morinville, A; Hoffert, C; Hubatsch, D; O'Donnell, D; Beaudet, A. Immunohistochemical distribution of delta opioid receptors in the rat central nervous system: evidence for somatodendritic labeling and antigen-specific cellular compartmentalization. *J. Comp. Neurol.*, 2001b 440, 65-84.

Cahill, CM; Morinville, A; Hoffert, C; O'Donnell, D; Beaudet, A. Up-regulation and trafficking of delta opioid receptor in a model of chronic inflammation: implications for pain control. *Pain,* 2003 101, 199-208.

Cahill, CM; Morinville, A; Lee, MC; Vincent, JP; Collier, B; Beaudet, A. Prolonged morphine treatment targets delta opioid receptors to neuronal plasma membranes and enhances delta-mediated antinociception. *J. Neurosci.,* 2001a 21, 7598-75607.

Cahill, CM; White, TD; Sawynok, J. Synergy between mu/delta-opioid receptors mediates adenosine release from spinal cord synaptosomes. *Eur J. Pharmacol.,* 1996 298, 45–49.

Caulfield, MP. Muscarinic receptors-characterization, coupling and function. *Pharmacol. Ther.,* 1993 58, 319-379.

Charles, AC; Mostovskaya, N; Asas, K; Evans, CJ; Dankovich, ML; Hales, TG. Coexpression of delta-opioid receptors with micro receptors in GH3 cells changes the functional response to micro agonists from inhibitory to excitatory. *Mol. Pharmacol.,* 2003 63, 89-95.

Chen, SR; Pan, HL. Activation of muscarinic receptors inhibits spinal dorsal horn projection neurons: role of GABAB receptors. *Neuroscience*, 2004 125, 141-148.

Chen, SR; Pan, HL. Blocking mu opioid receptors in the spinal cord prevents the analgesic action by subsequent systemic opioids. *Brain Res.*, 2006 1081, 119-125.

Chen, SR; Pan, HL. Spinal endogenous acetylcholine contributes to the analgesic effect of systemic morphine in rats. *Anesthesiology*, 2001 95, 525-530.

Chen, SR; Wess, J; Pan, HL. Functional activity of the M2 and M4 receptor subtypes in the spinal cord studied with muscarinic acetylcholine receptor knockout mice. *J. Pharmacol. Exp. Ther.,* 2005 313, 765-770.

Cichewicz, DL; Martin, ZL; Smith, FL; Welch, SP. Enhancement mu opioid antinociception by oral delta9-tetrahydrocannabinol: dose-response analysis and receptor identification. *J. Pharmacol. Exp. Ther.*, 1999 289, 859-867.

Cichewicz, DL. Synergistic interactions between cannabinoid and opioid analgesics. *Life Sci.*, 2004 74, 1317-1324.

Connor, M; Christie, MD. Opioid receptor signalling mechanisms. *Clin. Exp. Pharmacol. Physiol.*, 1999 26, 493-499.

Corchero, J; Avila, MA; Fuentes, JA; Manzanares, J. Delta-9-Tetrahydrocannabinol increases prodynorphin and proenkephalin gene expression in the spinal cord of the rat. *Life Sci.,* 1997 61, 39-43.

De Camilli, P; Jahn, R. Pathways to regulated exocytosis in neurons. *Annu. Rev. Physiol.,* 1990 52, 625-645.

De Vries, TJ; Van Vliet, BJ; Hogenboom, F; Wardeh, G; Van der Laan, JW; Mulder, AH; Schoffelmeer, AN. Effect of chronic prenatal morphine treatment of mu-opioid receptor-regulated adenylate cyclase activity and neurotransmitter release in rat brain slices. *Eur. J. Pharmacol.,* 1991 208, 97-104.

Dickenson, AH; Sullivan, AF; Knox, R; Zajac, JM; Roques, BP. Opioid receptor subtypes in the rat spinal cord: electrophysiological studies with mu- and delta-opioid receptor agonists in the control of nociception. *Brain Res.,* 1987 413, 36-44.

Dickenson, AH; Suzuki, R. Opioids in neuropathic pain: clues from animal studies. *Eur. J. Pain*, 2005 9, 113–116.

Dickenson, AH. Spinal cord pharmacology of pain. *Br. J. Anaesth.,* 1995 75, 193-200.

Doly, S; Fischer, J; Brisorgueil, MJ; Vergé, D; Conrath, M. Pre- and postsynaptic localization of the 5-HT7 receptor in rat dorsal spinal cord: immunocytochemical evidence. *J. Comp. Neurol.,* 2005 490, 256–269.

Duttaroy, A; Gomeza, J; Gan, JW; Siddiqui, N; Basile, AS; Harman, WD; Smith, PL; Felder, CC; Levey, AI; Wess, J. Evaluation of muscarinic agonist-induced analgesia in muscarinic acetylcholine receptor knockout mice. *Mol. Pharmacol.,* 2002 62, 1084-1093.

Edwards, RR. Individual differences in endogenous pain modulation as a risk factor for chronic pain. *Neurology,* 2005 65, 437–443.

Egan, TM; North, RA. Both mu and delta opiate receptors exist on the same neuron. *Science,* 1981 214, 923–924.

Elmes, SJ; Jhaveri, MD; Smart, D; Kendall, DA; Chapman, V. Cannabinoid CB2 receptor activation inhibits mechanically evoked responses of wide dynamic range dorsal horn neurons in naïve rats and in rat models of inflammatory and neuropathic pain. *Eur. J. Neurosci.,* 2004 20, 2311-2320.

Evans, CJ; Keith, DE Jr; Morrison, H; Magendzo, K; Edwards, RH. Cloning of a delta opioid receptor by functional expression. *Science,* 1992 258, 1952-1955.

Fairbanks, CA; Stone, LS; Kitto, KF; Nguyen, HO; Posthumus, IJ; Wilcox, GL. Alpha(2C)-Adrenergic receptors mediate spinal analgesia and adrenergic-opioid synergy. *J. Pharmacol. Exp. Ther.,* 2002 300, 282-290.

Fan, T; Varghese, G; Nguyen T; Tse, R; O'Dowd, BF; George, SR. A role for the distal carboxyl tails in generating the novel pharmacology and G protein activation profile of mu and delta opioid receptor hetero-oligomers. *J. Biol. Chem.*, 2005 280, 38478-38488.

Fields, TA; Casey, PJ. Signalling functions and biochemical properties of pertussis toxin-resistant G-proteins. *Biochem. J.,* 1997 321, 561-571.

Gendron, L; Esdaile, MJ; Mennicken, F; Pan, H; O'Donnell, D; Vincent, JP; Devi, LA; Cahill, CM; Stroh, T; Beaudet, A. Morphine priming in rats with chronic inflammation reveals a dichotomy between antihyperalgesic and antinociceptive properties of deltorphin. *Neuroscience,* 2007 144, 263-274.

George, SR; Fan, T; Xie, Z; Tse, R; Tam, V; Varghese, G; O'Dowd, BF. Oligomerization of mu- and delta-opioid receptors. Generation of novel functional properties. *J. Biol. Chem.,* 2000 275, 26128-26135.

George, SR; O'Dowd, BF; Lee, SP. G-protein-coupled receptor oligomerization and its potential for drug discovery. *Nat. Rev. Drug. Discov.,* 2002 1, 808-820.

Gomes, I; Gupta, A; Filipovska J; Szeto, HH; Pintar, JE; Devi, LA. A role for heterodimerization of mu and delta opiate receptors in enhancing morphine analgesia. *Proc. Natl. Acad. Sci. USA,* 2004 101, 5135-5139.

Gomes, I; Jordan, BA; Gupta, A; Trapaidze, N; Nagy, V; Devi, LA. Heterodimerization of mu and delta opioid receptors: A role in opiate synergy. *J. Neurosci.*, 2000 20, 1-5.

Grabow, TS; Hurley, RW; Banfor, PN; Hammond, DL. Supraspinal and spinal delta2 opioid receptor-mediated antinociceptive synergy is mediated by spinal alpha2 adrenoceptors. Pain, 1999 83, 47-55.

Guan, JS; Xu, ZZ; Gao, H; He, SQ; Ma, GQ; Sun, T; Wang, LH; Zhang, ZN; Lena, I; Kitchen, I; Elde, R; Zimmer, A; He, C; Pei, G; Bao, L; Zhang, X. Interaction with vesicle luminal protachykinin regulates surface expression of delta-opioid receptors and opioid analgesia. *Cell,* 2005 122, 619-631.

Guo, XH; Fairbanks, CA; Stone, LS; Loh, HH. DPDPE-UK14,304 synergy is retained in mu opioid receptor knockout mice. *Pain,* 2003 104, 209-217.

Gurevich, VV; Gurevich, EV. GPCR monomers and oligomers: it takes all kinds. *Trends Neurosci.,* 2008 31, 74-81.

Hague, C; Uberti, MA; Chen, Z; Hall, RA; Minneman, KP. Cell surface expression of alpha1D-adrenergic receptors is controlled by heterodimerization with alpha1B-adrenergic receptors. *J. Biol. Chem.,* 2004 279, 15541-15549.

Hojo, M; Sudo, Y; Ando, Y; Minami, K; Takada, M; Matsubara, T; Kanaide, M; Taniyama, K; Sumikawa, K; Uezono, Y. mu-Opioid receptor forms a functional heterodimer with cannabinoid CB1 receptor: electrophysiological and FRET assay analysis. *J. Pharmacol. Sci.,* 2008 108, 308-319.

Holdridge, SV; Cahill, CM. Spinal administration of a delta opioid receptor agonist attenuates hyperalgesia and allodynia in a rat model of neuropathic pain. *Eur. J. Pain,* 2007 11, 685–693.

Honda, K; Ando, S; Koga, K; Takano, Y. The spinal muscarinic receptor subtypes contribute to the morphine-induced antinociceptive effects in thermal stimulation in mice. *Neurosci. Lett.,* 2004 371, 235-238.

Hood, DD; Mallak, KA; James, RL; Tuttle, R; Eisenach, JC. Enhancement of analgesia from systemic opioid in humans by spinal cholinesterase inhibition. *J. Pharmacol. Exp. Ther.,* 1997 282, 86-92.

Howlett, AC; Qualy, JM; Khachatrian, LL. Involvement of Gi in the inhibition of adenylate cyclase by cannabimimetic drugs. *Mol. Pharmacol.,* 1986 29, 307-313.

Hoyer, D; Clarke, DE; Fozard, JR; Hartig, PR; Martin, GR; Mylecharane, EJ; Saxena, PR; Humphrey, PP. International Union of Pharmacology classification of receptors for 5-hydroxytryptamine (Serotonin). *Pharmacol. Rev.,* 1994 46, 157–203.

Huang, LY; Neher, E. Ca(2+)-dependent exocytosis in the somata of dorsal root ganglion neurons. *Neuron,* 1996 17, 135-145.

Ji, RR; Zhang, Q; Law, PY; Low, HH; Elde, R; Hokfelt, T. Expression of mu-, delta-, and kappa-opioid receptor-like immunoreactivities in rat dorsal root ganglia after carrageenan-induced inflammation. *J. Neurosci.,* 1995 15, 8156–8166.

Jordan, BA; Devi, LA. G-protein-coupled receptor heterodimerization modulates receptor function. *Nature,* 1999 399, 697-700.

Jung, LJ; Scheller, RH. Peptide processing and targeting in the neuronal secretory pathway. *Science,* 1991 251, 1330-1335.

Kayser, V; Guilbaud, G. Physiological relevance and time course of a tonic endogenous opioid modulation of nociceptive messages, based on the effects of naloxone in a rat model of localized hyperalgesic inflammation. *Brain Res.,* 1990 567, 197–203.

Keck, BJ; Stafinsky, JL; Uram, M; Crisp, T. A lack of supersensitivity to opioid receptor agonists following chronic spinal opioid receptor antagonist administration in the rat. *Gen. Pharmacol.,* 1995 26, 161–168.

Kelly, S; Jhaveri, MD; Sagar, DR; Kendall, DA; Chapman, V. Activation of peripheral cannabinoid CB1 receptors inhibits mechanically evoked responses of spinal neurons in noninflamed rats and rats with hindpaw inflammation. *Eur. J. Neurosci.,* 2003 18, 2239-2243.

Kidd, EJ; Laporte, AM; Langlois, X; Fattaccini, CM; Doyen, C; Lombard, MC; Gozlan, H; Hamon, M. 5-HT3 receptors in the rat central nervous system are mainly located on nerve fibres and terminals. *Brain Res.*, 1993 612, 289–298.

Kieffer, BL; Befort, K; Gaveriaux-Ruff, C; Hirth, CG. The delta-opioid receptor: isolation of a cDNA by expression cloning and pharmacological characterization. *Proc. Natl. Acad. Sci. USA*, 1992 89, 12048-12052.

Kim, H; Neubert, JK; San Miguel, A; Xu, K; Krishnaraju, RK; Iadarola, MJ; Goldman, D; Dionne, RA. Genetic influence on variability in human acute experimental pain sensitivity associated with gender, ethnicity and psychological temperament. *Pain,* 2004 109, 488-496.

Kohno, T; Kumamoto, E; Higashi, H; Shimoji, K; Yoshimura, M. Actions of opioids on excitatory and inhibitory transmission in substantia gelatinosa of adult rat spinal cord. *J. Physiol.,* 1999 518, 803-813.

Kovelowski, CJ; Bian, D; Hruby, VJ; Lai, J; Ossipov, MH; Porreca, F. Selective opioid delta agonists elicit antinociceptive supraspinal/spinal synergy in the rat. *Brain Res.,* 1999 843, 12–17.

Law, PY; Erickson-Herbrandson, LJ; Zha, QQ; Solberg, J; Chu, J; Sarre, A; Loh, HH. Heterodimerization of mu- and delta-opioid receptors occurs at the cell surface only and requires receptor-G protein interactions. *J. Biol. Chem.*, 2005 280, 11152-11164.

Law, PY; Wong, YH; Loh, HH. Molecular mechanisms and regulation of opioid receptor signaling. *Annu. Rev. Pharmacol. Toxicol.,* 2000 40, 389-430.

Leskelä, TT; Markkanen, PM; Alahuhta, IA; Tuusa, JT; Petäjä-Repo, UE. Phe27Cys polymorphism alters the maturation and subcellular localization of the human delta opioid receptor. *Traffic*, 2009 10, 116-129.

Levine, JD; Gordon, NC; Jones, RT; Fields, HL. The narcotic antagonist naloxone enhances clinical pain. *Nature,* 1977 272, 826–827.

Li, DP; Chen, SR; Pan, YZ; Levey, AI; Pan, HL. Role of presynaptic muscarinic and GABA(B) receptors in spinal glutamate release and cholinergic analgesia in rats. *J. Physiol.*, 2002 543, 807-818.

MacDonald, E; Kobilka, BK; Scheinin, M. Gene targeting--homing in on alpha 2-adrenoceptor-subtype function. *Trends Pharmacol. Sci.,* 1997 18, 211-219.

Malcangio, M; Bowery, NG. Gamma-aminobutyric acidB, but not gamma-aminobutyric acidA receptor activation, inhibits electrically evoked substance P-like immunoreactivity release from the rat spinal cord in vitro. *J. Pharmacol. Exp. Ther.,* 1993 266, 1490–1496.

Malmberg, AB; Yaksh, TL. Isobolographic and dose–response analyses of the interaction between intrathecal mu and delta agonists: effects of naltrindole and its benzofuran analog (NTB). *J. Pharmacol. Exp. Ther.,* 1992 263, 264–275.

Margeta-Mitrovic, M; Jan, YN; Jan, LY. A trafficking checkpoint controls GABA(B) receptor heterodimerization. *Neuron,* 2000 27, 97-106.

Marlier, L; Teilhac, JR; Cerruti, C; Privat, A. Autoradiographic mapping of 5-HT1, 5-HT1A, 5-HT1B and 5-HT2 receptors in the rat spinal cord. *Brain Res.,* 1991 550, 15–23.

Marvizon, JC; Grady, EF; Stefani, E; Bunnett, NW; Mayer, EA. Substance P release in the dorsal horn assessed by receptor internalization: NMDA receptors counteract a tonic inhibition by GABA(B) receptors. *Eur. J. Neurosci.*, 1999 11, 417–426.

Matsumoto, I; Combs, MR; Jones, DJ. Characterization of 5-hydroxytryptamine1B receptors in rat spinal cord via [125I] iodocyanopindolol binding and inhibition of [3H]-5-hydroxytryptamine release. *J. Pharmacol. Exp. Ther.*, 1992 260, 614–626.

Mika, J; Przewlocki, R; Przewlocka, B. The role of delta-opioid receptor. *Eur. J. Pharmacol.*, 2001 415, 31-37.

Millan, MJ. Descending control of pain. *Prog. Neurobiol.*, 2002 66, 355-474.

Millan, MJ. The induction of pain: an integrative review. *Prog. Neurobiol.*, 1999 57, 1-164.

Milligan, G. G protein-coupled receptor dimerization: function and ligand pharmacology. *Mol. Pharmacol.*, 2004 66, 1-7.

Mizoguchi, H; Narita, M; Nagase, H; Tseng, LF. Antisense oligodeoxynucleotide to a delta-opioid receptor blocks the antinociception induced by cold water swimming. *Regul. Pept.*, 1995 59, 255–259.

Nadal, X; Baños, JE; Kieffer, BL; Maldonado, R. Neuropathic pain is enhanced in delta-opioid receptor knockout mice. *Eur. J. Neurosci.*, 2006 23, 830-834.

Nichols, DE; Nichols, CD. Serotonin receptors. *Chem. Rev.*, 2008 108, 1614-1641.

Overland, AC; Kitto, KF; Chabot-Doré, AJ; Rothwell, PE; Fairbanks, CA; Stone, LS; Wilcox, GL. Protein kinase C mediates the synergistic interaction between agonists acting at alpha2-adrenergic and delta-opioid receptors in spinal cord. *J. Neurosci.*, 2009 29, 13264-13273.

Pan, HL; Wu, ZZ; Zhou, HY; Chen, SR; Zhang, HM; Li, DP. Modulation of pain transmission by G-protein-coupled receptors. *Pharmacol. Ther.*, 2008 117, 141-161.

Philipp, M; Brede, M; Hein, L. Physiological significance of alpha(2)-adrenergic receptor subtype diversity: one receptor is not enough. *Am. J. Physiol. Regul. Integr. Comp. Physiol.*, 2002 283, 287-295.

Porreca, F; Ossipov, MH; Gebhart, GF. Chronic pain and medullary descending facilitation. *Trends Neurosci.*, 2002 25, 319–325.

Reche, I; Fuentes, JA; Ruiz-Gayo, M. Potentiation of delta 9-tetrahydrocannabinol-induced analgesia by morphine in mice: involvement of mu- and kappa-opioid receptors. *Eur. J. Pharmacol.*, 1996 318, 11-16.

Riedl, MS; Schnell, SA; Overland, AC; Chabot-Doré, AJ; Taylor, AM; Ribeiro-da-Silva, A; Elde, RP; Wilcox, GL; Stone, LS. Coexpression of alpha 2A-adrenergic and delta-opioid receptors in substance P-containing terminals in rat dorsal horn. *J. Comp. Neurol.*, 2009 513, 385-398.

Rizzo, MA; Springer, GH; Granada, B; Piston, DW. An improved cyan fluorescent protein variant useful for FRET. *Nat. Biotechnol.*, 2004 22, 445-449.

Roerig, SC; Lei, S; Kitto, K; Hylden, JK; Wilcox, GL. Spinal interactions between opioid and noradrenergic agonists in mice: multiplicativity involves delta and alpha-2 receptors. *J. Pharmacol. Exp. Ther.*, 1992 262, 365-374.

Rubino, T; Viganò, D; Massi, P; Parolaro, D. Changes in the cannabinoid receptor binding, G protein coupling, and cyclic AMP cascade in the CNS of rats tolerant to and dependent on the synthetic cannabinoid compound CP55,940. *J. Neurochem.*, 2000 75, 2080-2086.

Saeki, S; Yaksh, TL. Suppression of nociceptive responses by spinal mu opioid agonists: effects of stimulus intensity and agonist efficacy. *Anesth. Analg.*, 1993 77, 265–274.

Sagar, DR; Kelly, S; Millns, PJ; O'Shaughnessey, CT; Kendall, DA; Chapman, V. Inhibitory effects of CB1 and CB2 receptor agonists on responses of DRG neurons and dorsal horn neurons in neuropathic rats. *Eur. J. Neurosci.*, 2005 22, 371-379.

Salahpour, A; Angers, S; Bouvier, M. Functional significance of oligomerization of G-protein-coupled receptors. *Trends Endocrinol. Metab.*, 2000 11, 163-168.

Salio, C; Fischer, J; Franzoni, MF; Conrath, M. Pre- and postsynaptic localizations of the CB1 cannabinoid receptor in the dorsal horn of the rat spinal cord. *Neuroscience,* 2002 110, 755-764.

Salio, C; Fischer, J; Franzoni, MF; Mackie, K; Kaneko, T; Conrath, M. CB1-cannabinoid and mu-opioid receptor co-localization on postsynaptic target in the rat dorsal horn. *Neuroreport,* 2001 12, 3689-3692.

Shapira, M; Vogel, Z; Sarne, Y. Opioid and cannabinoid receptors share a common pool of GTP-binding proteins in cotransfected cells, but not in cells which endogenously coexpress the receptors. *Cell Mol. Neurobiol.,* 2000 20, 291-304.

Stevens, CW; Kajander, KC; Bennett, GJ; Seybold, VS. Bilateral and differential changes in spinal mu, delta and kappa opioid binding in rats with a painful, unilateral neuropathy. *Pain,* 1991 46, 315–326.

Stone, LS; MacMillan, LB; Kitto, KF; Limbird, LE; Wilcox, GL. The alpha2a adrenergic receptor subtype mediates spinal analgesia evoked by alpha2 agonists and is necessary for spinal adrenergic-opioid synergy. *J. Neurosci.,* 1997 17, 7157-7165.

Stone, LS; Vulchanova, L; Riedl, MS; Williams, FG; Wilcox, GL; Elde, R. Effects of peripheral nerve injury on delta opioid receptor (DOR) immunoreactivity in the rat spinal cord. *Neurosci. Lett.*, 2004 361, 208–211.

Sullivan, AF; Dickenson, AH; Roques, BP. Delta-opioid mediated inhibitions of acute and prolonged noxious-evoked responses in rat dorsal horn neurones. *Br. J. Pharmacol.,* 1989 98, 1039-1049.

Suzuki, R; Morcuende, S; Webber, M; Hunt, SP; Dickenson, AH. Superficial NK1-expressing neurons control spinal excitability through activation of descending pathways. *Nat. Neurosci.*, 2002 5, 1319–1326.

Tanabe, M; Murakami, H; Honda, M; Ono, H. Gabapentin depresses C-fiber-evoked field potentials in rat spinal dorsal horn only after induction of long-term potentiation. *Exp. Neurol.,* 2006 202, 280–286.

Taylor, BK Spinal inhibitory neurotransmission in neuropathic pain. *Curr. Pain Headache. Rep.*, 2009 13, 208-214.

Terrillon, S; Durroux, T; Mouillac, B; Breit, A; Ayoub, MA; Taulan, M; Jockers, R; Barberis, C; Bouvier, M. Oxytocin and vasopressin V1a and V2 receptors form constitutive homo- and heterodimers during biosynthesis. *Mol. Endocrinol.,* 2003 17, 677-691.

Traynor, J; Elliot, J. Delta-opioid receptor subtypes and cross talk with mureceptors. *Trends Pharmacol. Sci.,* 1993 14, 84–86.

Tsou, K; Brown, S; Sañudo-Peña, MC; Mackie, K; Walker, JM. Immunohistochemical distribution of cannabinoid CB1 receptors in the rat central nervous system. *Neuroscience,* 1998 83, 393-411.

Walwyn, W; John, S; Maga, M; Evans, CJ; Hales, TG. Delta receptors are required for full inhibitory coupling of mu-receptors to voltage-dependent Ca(2+) channels in dorsal root ganglion neurons. *Mol. Pharmacol.*, 2009 76, 134-143.

Wang, HB; Guan, JS; Bao, L; Zhang, X. Distinct subcellular distribution of delta-opioid receptor fused with various tags in PC12 cells. *Neurochem. Res.,* 2008 33, 2028-2034.

Wang, W; Wu, SX; Wang, YY; Liu, XY; Li, YQ. 5-hydroxytryptamine 1A receptor is involved in the bee venom induced inflammatory pain. *Pain,* 2003 106, 135–142.

Welch, SP; Stevens, DL. Antinociceptive activity of intrathecally administered cannabinoids alone, and in combination with morphine, in mice. *J. Pharmacol. Exp. Ther.,* 1992 262, 10-18.

Wess, J; Duttaroy, A; Gomeza, J; Zhang, W; Yamada, M; Felder, CC; Bernardini, N; Reeh, PW. Muscarinic receptor subtypes mediating central and peripheral antinociception studied with muscarinic receptor knockout mice: a review. *Life Sci.,* 2003 72, 2047-2054.

Woolf, CJ; Salter, MW. Neuronal plasticity: increasing the gain in pain. *Science*, 2000 288, 1765–1769.

Wu, S; Zhu, M; Wang, W; Wang, Y; Li, Y; Yew, DT. Changes of the expression of 5-HT receptor subtype mRNAs in rat dorsal root ganglion by complete Freund's adjuvant-induced inflammation. *Neurosci. Lett.*, 2001 307, 183–186.

Xie, Z; Lee, SP; O'Dowd, BF; George, SR. Serotonin 5-HT1B and 5-HT1D receptors form homodimers when expressed alone and heterodimers when co-expressed. *FEBS Lett.*, 1999 456, 63-67.

Yoshimura, M; Furue, H. Mechanisms for the anti-nociceptive actions of the descending noradrenergic and serotonergic systems in the spinal cord. *J. Pharmacol. Sci.*, 2006 101, 107-117.

Zhang, H; Kranzler, HR; Yang, BZ; Luo, X; Gelernter, J. The OPRD1 and OPRK1 loci in alcohol or drug dependence: OPRD1 variation modulates substance dependence risk. *Mol. Psychiatry.,* 2008 13, 531-543.

Zhang, X; Bao, L; Arvidsson, U; Elde, R; Hökfelt T. Localization and regulation of the delta-opioid receptor in dorsal root ganglia and spinal cord of the rat and monkey: evidence for association with the membrane of large dense-core vesicles. *Neuroscience*, 1998 82, 1225-1242.

Zhuo, M; Gebhart, GF. Spinal serotonin receptors mediate descending facilitation of a nociceptive reflex from the nuclei reticularis gigantocellularis and gigantocellularis pars alpha in the rat. *Brain Res.*, 1991 550, 35-48.

Zimmermann, M. Pathobiology of neuropathic pain. *Eur. J. Pharmacol.,* 2001 429, 23–37.

In: Opioids: Pharmacology, Clinical Uses and Adverse Effects ISBN 978-1-61942-101-1
Editors: Djavakhi Tvildiani and Kakha Gegechkori

Chapter 5

OPIOIDS: PHARMACOLOGY, CLINICAL USES AND ADVERSE EFFECTS

Robert Taylor Jr.[1], Joseph V. Pergolizzi Jr.[2], Robert B. Raffa[3] and Edmundo Muniz[4]

[1]NEMA Research, Naples, FL, US

[2]Department of Medicine, Johns Hopkins University, Baltimore, MD, Department of Pharmacology, Temple University School of Medicine, Philadelphia, PA, US, and Department of Anesthesiology, Georgetown University School of Medicine, Washington, DC, US

[3]Department of Pharmaceutical Sciences, Temple University School of Pharmacy, Philadelphia, PA, US

[4]Tigris Pharmaceuticals, Bonita Springs, FL, US

ABSTRACT

This chapter presents a concise overview of the pharmacology, clinical uses, and adverse effects of morphine-like drugs ('opioids'). Morphine, a natural product whose beneficial therapeutic use was discovered serendipitously thousands of years ago, remains the 'gold standard' for the relief of moderate to severe pain. Following the elucidation of morphine's chemical structure at the beginning of the 19th century and subsequent extensive design, synthesis, and testing of chemical analogs by pharmaceutical and academic laboratories, today there are multiple opioids available to thc clinician. Although each is morphine-like and shares certain fundamental characteristics with morphine, they each have particular features, the nuances of which influence their clinical use and usefulness.

1. INTRODUCTION

Opioids are among the oldest and most enduring substances used for the management of moderate to severe pain and other medical problems, such as diarrhea. It is now known that the properties of the naturally occurring opioids ('opiates', primarily morphine and codeine) and the related endogenous opioid-like peptides (e.g., endorphins, enkephalins, dynorphins) and synthetic chemical substances can be attributed to action at the receptors to which they bind within the central and peripheral nervous systems. There are three major opioid receptor types, each identified and named based on an agonist that binds with relative selectivity: mu (morphine); kappa (ketocyclazocine); and delta ([D-Ala^2, D-Leu^5]-enkephalin). Opioid receptors are widely distributed throughout the central and peripheral nervous systems and to variable extent can be up-regulated under certain conditions. Upon agonist binding, all three opioid receptor types mediate the therapeutic and adverse effects of opioids to an extent dictated by the receptor type-selectivity of the agonist.

The clinical application of opioids has included extensive utilization in areas of acute- and postoperative-type pain settings. Opioid analgesics are currently being used, or evaluated for use, in cancer, non-cancer (e.g., rheumatoid arthritis), and neuropathic pain conditions. The adverse event profile of opioid treatment varies depending on the particular opioid, but some well known common side effects include constipation, nausea, vomiting, sedation, mental clouding, impaired psychomotor function, and respiratory depression at high doses. Other side effects may also include immunosuppression and endocrine alterations. Because of this profile, opioid use requires a well thought out treatment plan of action before prescribing.

The aging of the population will create an increase in the incidence and prevalence of pain. This significant demographic shift will create larger and more complicated demands for the appropriate use of all pain medications, including opioids. Challenges in pain management will arise in the elderly because of the physiological changes that occur during aging. These include changes in aspects of pain perception, cognitive impairment or compliance, changes in physiology that alter drug pharmacokinetic profiles, in addition to having a wide range of pain of varying etiologies. In addition, elderly patients are more likely to have comorbidities that require multiple medications (polypharmacy), thus increasing the chance of drug-drug interactions.

Mu-opioid analgesic agonists are Schedule II controlled substances in the United States. Such drugs are sought by drug abusers and people with addiction disorders. Diversion of Schedule II products is an act subject to criminal penalty. Mu-opioids, legal or illicit, can be abused in a manner similar. This should be considered when prescribing or dispensing opioids in situations where the physician or pharmacist is concerned about an increased risk of misuse and abuse. Concerns about abuse and addiction should not prevent the proper management of pain. However, all patients treated with mu-opioid agonists require careful monitoring for signs of abuse and addiction, since use of mu-opioid analgesic products carry the risk of addiction even under appropriate medical use. Therefore, appropriate patient selection and utilization of universal opioid precautions, along with an integrated drug compliance monitoring, are necessary when prescribing or dispensing this class of compounds because of documented cases of nonmedical use, abuse, misuse, and diversion.

When used as indicated, and with appropriate and judicious vigilance for patients who might be particularly at risk for adverse effects or abuse, opioid analgesics provide generally safe and efficacious drugs for the management of moderate to severe pain arising from multiple etiologies.

2. General Overview of Opioid Pharmacology

2.1. Pharmacodynamics (PD)

Knowledge of the pharmacological properties of extracts of the opium poppy plant *Papaver somniferum* can be traced back at least 8000 years to a Sumerian ideogram [1]. Already by the 2nd century BC, Arabs, Greeks, and Romans described the therapeutic use and adverse effects of the extracts [2]. In 1805, Friederich Wilhelm Sertürner, an apothecary's assistant in Hanover, Germany, isolated and purified morphine from the opium plant [3]. He named it for the Greek god of dreams and sleep, Morpheus. Following optimization of the extraction process by the Parisian pharmacist Pierre-Jean Robiquet, morphine was soon promoted as a commercial product. It was available in London by 1821 and wholesale production by the German pharmacist Heinrich Emanuel Merck began a few years later[4].

In addition to morphine, other naturally occurring alkaloids obtained from the resin of the opium poppy plant ('opiates') include codeine, thebaine, noscapine, and papaverine. 'Semi-synthetic' opioids, which are derived from natural opiates and share a similar chemical structure, include hydrocodone, oxycodone, oxymorphone, hydromorphone, buprenorphine, and diacetylmorphine (heroin). 'Fully synthetic' opioids include methadone, fentanyl, pethidine, tramadol, dextropropoxyphene (no longer available in the US) and many others.

The prototypical opioid structure is that of morphine. The morphine template consists of five interlocked rings with attached functional groups [5]. The chemical properties of the particular functional groups determine each opioid's individual pharmacologic properties. Although not all of the known opioids strickly conform to this standard structure, they must meet the conformational requirements to bind to and activate opioid receptors in a similar manner.

In the early 1970s it was discovered that the body produces its own endogenous opioids for use as neurotransmitters or neuromodulators [6]. The endogenous opioids include endorphins, enkephalins, dynorphins, and endomorphins. Endogenous opioids participate in the regulation of bodily functions such as hunger, thirst, mood control, immune response, and reactions to painful stimuli [7]. Endorphins (chiefly β-endorphin) are derived from the large precursor molecule proopiomelanocortin (POMC), are localized primarily in the pituitary and hypothalamus, and are known to have analgesic activity [8]. Enkephalins include several compounds derived from a large proenkephalin molecule (also called proenkephalin A), are distributed throughout the central nervous system, and modulate neurotransmitter release [8]. Dynorphins are derived from a prodynorphin molecule (also called proenkephalin B) and have a similar distribution as the enkephalins. It is also known that all opioids (endogenous, naturally-derived, semi-synthetic, and synthetic) interact with specific receptors [8].

The general structure of all opioid receptors resembles that of the G protein-coupled receptors (GPCRs). They contain an extracellular *N*-terminal domain and an intracellular *C*-terminal domain, joined in the middle by seven transmembrane domains[9, 10]. The mu, delta, and kappa receptors share approximately 60% homology, with the greatest similarity within their transmembrane helical domains and the greatest diversity within the *N* and *C* termini and the extracellular loops [11]. Other conserved amino acids include two conserved cysteine residues that reside in the first and second extracellular loops and modified Asn-linked glycosyl chains at various sites in their *N*-terminal domains [9].

Most of the opioid analgesics in current clinical use bind primarily to the mu opioid receptor (with present preferred terminology MOR)[10]. A majority of MORs are located within the central nervous system and are concentrated within the brain (laminae III and IV of the cortex, medial thalamus, periaqueductal gray) and the spinal cord (substantia gelatinosa) [4]. In addition, MORs are also located in peripheral tissues, in particular the gastrointestinal tract [12]. Different aspects of opioid pharmacology have been attributed to one or another MOR subtype [4, 10]. Subtypes of each of the three major opioid receptor types have been postulated, but their contributions to the therapeutic or adverse effects of opioids have not been fully delineated and are beyond the scope of the present overview. Opioid agonists inhibit presynaptic influx of Ca^{2+} and enhance postsynaptic efflux of K^{+}. The former action inhibits the release of neurotransmitters thought to be involved in the transmission of pain signals; the latter hyperpolarizes the cell, making it less responsive to a pain signal [13] (Figure. 1).

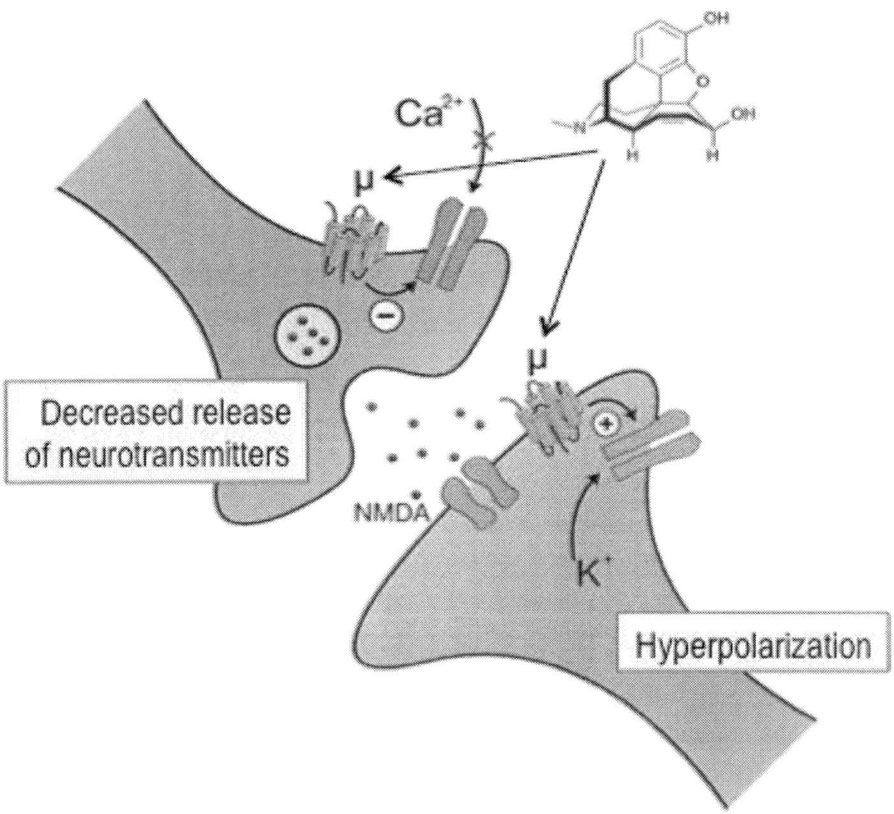

Figure 1.

Opioid antagonists, such as naloxone and naltrexone, compete with opioids at opioid receptor sites [14]. Thus they can be used to reverse opioid receptor-mediated adverse effects such as respiratory depression [15]. They are also used for various aspects of the management of opioid abuse [15].

Agonist-antagonist (also known as mixed agonist-antagonist) opioids are agonists at one opioid receptor subtype and antagonists at another receptor subtype (e.g. butorphanol, dezocine, nalbuphine, pentazocine) [4, 14]. These drugs can be used as analgesics, but normally have a ceiling to their analgesic effect, thus making their use in the general population limited. Increasing the dosage beyond a certain level will generally only yield greater side effects [4].

2.2. Pharmacokinetics

Opioids are generally well absorbed by almost all routes of administration, both peripheral (e.g., subcutaneous, intramuscular, rectal, inhalational) and central (e.g., intrathecal) [16, 17]. The bioavailability and pharmacologic effects following oral administration differs greatly for each opioid due to differences in first pass metabolism [17].

The volume of distribution and percent of protein binding varies for each of the opioids. Absorption into tissues depends mainly on the hydrophobicity of the compounds. So for example, morphine (more hydrophilic) slowly absorbs into adipose tissue compared to fentanyl (more hydrophobic). Hydrophobicity also is a major determinant in an opioid's ability to cross the blood brain barrier. More hydrophilic opioids such as morphine do not pass the barrier rapidly [18], whereas more hydrophobic opioids such as heroin or fentanyl pass more rapidly [18].

Most opioids are primarily metabolized in the liver, undergoing Phase 1 and/or Phase 2 type biotransformation reactions [14]. The Phase 1 reactions are catalyzed by cytochrome P450 enzymes, in particular the CYP3A4 and CYP2D6 isozymes, but CYP2B6, CYP2C8, CYP2C19, and CYP2C9 can also contribute. Phase 2 metabolism consists primarily of conjugation reactions, specifically glucuronidation, catalyzed mainly by the UGT2B7 enzyme [14, 19].

Drug-drug interactions can occur with other drugs that are metabolized through the same metabolic pathways as are the opioids or with drugs that up- or down-regulate these enzymes [19].

Opioids are primarily excreted in the urine. Dosage adjustment is generally needed for patients with reduced renal function [20].

3. Clinical Uses

3.1. Analgesia

Opioids are generally known for their ability to treat moderate to severe pain, both in the acute [21] and chronic (cancer, non-cancer, neuropathic) pain settings [22-25]. Painful and noxious stimuli signals are transmitted to the spinal cord and eventually to the brain for processing. Opioid receptors are abundant throughout the central nervous system, located presynaptically and postsynaptically on neurons in the spinal cord in addition to the various parts of the brain (thalamus, mid-brain, medulla). Opioids generally block the nociceptive pain signals transmitted by both Aδ and C fibers to the central nervous system [26]. Agonist binding to opioid receptors on the presynaptic side of the neuron elicit an inhibitory response, attenuating neurotransmitter release to the second order neuron [26]. In addition, opioids hyperpolarize the postsynaptic neuron reducing the responsiveness to the first order neuron.

3.2. Other Uses

3.2.1. Cough Suppressant

Cough is a common, and at times medically serious symptom associated with infections of the upper and lower airway, asthma and COPD, lung cancer or lung metastases, interstitial pulmonary processes (such as lymphangitic tumor spread or pulmonary edema), gastroesophageal reflux, aspiration, and drugs [27, 28]. Severe cough can lead to dyspnea, nausea/vomiting, sleep impairment, and chest and throat pain [28]. Opioids are effective cough suppressors and are thought to work by suppressing the brainstem cough center through mu and kappa opioid receptor agonism. All opioid analgesics have some anti-tussive activity, but they have different potencies and efficacies and some, such as codeine and hydrocodone, are more popular than others.

3.2.2. Anti-diarrheal

Bacterial or viral infections, food intolerances, parasites, intestinal disease, bowel disorders, surgery, or reactions to medications are just some of the causes that can disrupt the gastrointestinal tract (GI) and lead to diarrhea. Symptoms of diarrhea normally include cramping, abdominal pain, bloating, and nausea. If left untreated, diarrhea can cause excessive weight loss, fevers, and intestinal damage. MOR are located in the gastrointestinal tract and agonist binding results in prolongation of GI transit time, which in turn can help reduce daily fecal volume, increase the viscosity and bulk density, and diminish the loss of fluids and electrolytes [29].

3.2.3. Use in Children and the Elderly

The prevalence and incidence of acute and chronic pain in children has been increasingly recognized and proper techniques and medications have been adapted from adult experiences [30]. Opioid use has been limited in children due to their potential for addiction and abuse, but their analgesic and side effects are similar to that experienced in adults. Codeine may be used for acute and chronic pain, but its variability in conversion to morphine in this patient population makes it an unreliable analgesic [31]. Morphine is the most frequently prescribed and studied opioid in children for both acute and chronic pain [32]. The slow release formulations of morphine are generally chosen for its safety and the length of analgesia achieved. Other opioids that have been used successfully include fentanyl and methadone [30, 33]. Both methadone and the transdermal fentanyl patch are a good, safe alternative for children requiring long acting and/or strong opioid therapy over an extended period of time [30]. Similar to adults, all opioids can potentially cause the same range of side effects including sedation, nausea/vomiting, pruritis, and respiratory depression. In addition, children can develop tolerance to opioids and in many opioid switching has been shown to be quite successful in the pediatric population [34].

Changes in body physiology, pain perception, and cognitive function are hurdles that are encountered when prescribing opioids to the elderly [35]. Renal and hepatic decline associated with aging can increase the half-life of many opioids (buprenorphine for example) and their metabolites, leading to prolonged analgesia and side effects [35]. Neurotoxicity may develop in the elderly population during long-term opioid use or in patients that have reduced renal function. They may experience hallucinations, confusion or even decline of alertness, which in turn may lead to an increase chance of bone fractures associated with falling. In addition, opioid-induced constipation can be exacerbated in the elderly. Many studies comparing the efficacy and tolerability of opioids in the elderly have been conducted. Generally, the elderly respond just as well as their younger counterparts.

4. Specific Agents

4.1. Morphine

Morphine is the prototypical mu receptor opiate agonist and the "gold standard" to which all other opioids are compared. The versatility by which morphine can be administered (IV, IM, IA, epidural, oral) has given physicians the ability to provide analgesia in a variety of pain conditions including both acute and chronic pain in addition to acting as an anti-diarrheal medication. Along with its therapeutic effects, morphine can produce nausea, vomiting, drowsiness, constipation, respiratory depression, changes in mood, and alterations of the endocrine and autonomic nervous systems. Both the analgesic and side effect profile of morphine may be influenced by its phase 2 metabolites morphine-6-glucoronide (analgesia) and morphine-3-glucoronide (adverse effects). The clinical profile of morphine is encompassed in the summary of opioid effects described above. Despite its side effects and abuse potential, morphine remains the standard of care for many types of pain [36-41].

4.2. Codeine

Codeine is used primarily as an analgesic for mild to moderate acute pain in addition to acting as an anti-diarrheal and cough suppressant [14]. It is an unresolved question whether codeine lacks the intrinsic activity to treat more severe pains or whether such use is limited by adverse effects and the availability of better alternatives. The analgesic and side effect profile of codeine most likely is the result of the Phase 1 conversion catalyzed by CYP2D6 into morphine [14]. This conversion is of particular importance in patients with genetic polymorphisms in CYP2D6 who are slow (low effect) or rapid (excess effect) metabolizers [14].

4.3. Dihydrocodeine

Dihydrocodeine is similar in structure to codeine (a phenanthrene) and has similar pharmacologic effects [42].

4.4. Fentanyl

Fentanyl, like the related alfentanil, remifentanil, and sufentanil, is a potent synthetic MOR agonist. Fentanyl use has mainly been for palliative and chronic pain, but has also been prescribed for breakthrough pain. Its high lipid solubility, which allows it to pass the blood brain barrier, makes it a prime candidate for transdermal and buccal delivery. Fentanyl undergoes first pass metabolism primarily via CYP3A4-catalyzed oxidative *N*-dealkylation to norfentanyl and other inactive metabolites and is eliminated primarily through the renal system [43].

4.5. Hydrocodone

Hydrocodone (dihydrocodeinone) is a semi-synthetic opioid agonist that has a similar structure to codeine (phenanthrene) and produces similar effects. Although it primarily acts at MOR, it also has weak agonist binding at delta and kappa opioid receptors. CYP2D6 and CYP3A4 catalyze the conversion of hydrocodone into hydromorphone, which is a more potent analgesic, and norhydrocodone. Hydrocodone has been marketed for both analgesia and as a cough suppressant, either alone or in combination with other analgesics such as acetaminophen, ibuprofen, or aspirin [44, 45].

4.6. Hydromorphone

Hydromorphone is a semi-synthetic, hydrogenated ketone of morphine with MOR agonist binding affinity [14]. Hydromorphone is approximately 3 to 4 times more potent than morphine as an analgesic for moderate to severe pain, has a much faster action of onset and presents many of the same side effects of other opioids. In addition to its analgesic properties, hydromorphone acts at the cough center in the medulla and thus is widely prescribed as a second or third line antitussive for cases of dry, painful, paroxysmal coughing [14]. The high lipid solubility allows for its rapid absorption from the gastrointestinal tract and thus is largely metabolized in first pass Phase 2 metabolism by glucuronidation, forming the main metabolite hydromorphone-6-glucoronide. Being mainly excreted by the renal system, patients with renal insufficiency should be titrated carefully because accumulation of hydromorphone and metabolites is linked to causing myoclonus, agitation, and seizures [46].

4.7. Oxycodone

Oxycodone is a synthetic opioid structurally similar to that of codeine and hydrocodone (phenanthrenes), with agonist activity on the mu, delta and kappa receptors. Indications for oxycodone are for moderate to severe pain. It is formulated as a single ingredient or with other analgesics including acetaminophen, ibuprofen, and aspirin. Similar to other opioids, the effects of oxycodone include euphoria, analgesia, sedation, relaxation, respiratory depression, constipation, papillary constriction, and cough suppression. Oxycodone undergoes metabolism by CYP2D6 in the liver, which forms the analgesic metabolites oxymorphone and noroxycodone, and is mainly excreted by the kidneys [47].

4.8. Oxymorphone

Produced from the natural opiate thebaine, oxymorphone is a semi-synthetic 6-keto opioid agonist. Oxymorphone is indicated for the relief of moderate to severe pain, chronic pain, breakthrough pain and it is used as a preoperative medication to alleviate apprehension and maintain anesthesia. Oxymorphone undergoes phase 2 metabolism to a glucuronide, thus reducing risk for drug drug interactions associated with the CYP450 system [48].

4.9. Buprenorphine

Buprenorphine is a thebaine derivative that in addition to use as an analgesic is indicated as an alternative to methadone for management of opioid addiction. It has been classified as a partial agonist at MOR, as well as a weak antagonist at the kappa opioid receptor. The oral bioavailability of buprenorphine is low due to extensive first pass hepatic metabolism, in which buprenorphine is demethylated to form the primary metabolite norbuprenorphine. Other metabolites are formed through CYP3A4 as well as UGT 1A3 and UGT2B7 pathways. Buprenorphine's strong lipophilicity allows it to be administered in many ways including IV, IM, IA, sublinigual, and by transdermal patches, making it versatile for many pain conditions [49, 50].

4.10. Levorphanol

Levorphanol tartrate is a potent synthetic opioid agonist used to treat severe pain [10]. Levorphanol is 4 to 8 times as potent as morphine, has a longer half-life than morphine, and has stronger affinity for mu, delta, and kappa opioid receptors than morphine. The longer duration of analgesia makes it useful in palliation of chronic pain and similar conditions. In addition, it also has NMDA antagonist properties, making it useful in neuropathic pain conditions. It is extensively metabolized in the liver by Phase 2 metabolism and is eliminated as the glucuronide metabolite.

4.11. Meperidine

Meperidine, otherwise known as pethidine,is a rapid acting synthetic opioid analgesic. Acting primarily as a kappa opioid receptor agonist, meperidine is indicated for the treatment of moderate to severe pain; however, its use for chronic pain is limited due to stimulating effects of the dopamine and norepinephrine transporters. Meperidine is metabolized in the liver via the cytochrome P450 system (CYP2B6, CYP3A4, CYP2D6, CYP1A2, CYP2C19) and undergoes hydrolysis to meperidinic acid followed by partial conjugation with glucuronic acid. *N*-demethylation leads to normeperidine, which has neurotoxic side effects that can lead to CNS hyperexcitablitiy, convulsions, seizures, delirium, and dysphoria. Normeperidine concentrations can build up in patients with renal impairment [51].

4.12. Methadone

Methadone is a synthetic opioid agonist with multiple indications including relief of severe pain, detoxification treatment of opioid addiction, and maintenance treatment of opioid addiction [52]. In addition to its MOR binding, methadone acts as an NMDA receptor antagonist, making it potentially useful for the prevention of opioid tolerance and treatment of neuropathic pain. Methadone is metabolized in the liver by the cytochrome P450 system (CYP2B6, CYP2C19, CYP2D6, etc) with a half-life of 8 to 60 hours [10]. Metabolic breakdown of methadone does not create active analgesic metabolites, thus dosing can be unaffected in patients with hepatic disease. Unlike many other opioids, methadone has been found to generate QT interval prolongation due to its interaction with voltage-gated potassium channels in the myocardium [53]. Therefore, caution should be taken when administered to patients on additional QT prolonging therapies.

4.13. Tramadol

Tramadol is a synthetic mixed opioid/nonopioid analgesic that has weak MOR agonist activity coupled with inhibition of neuronal reuptake of serotonin and norepinephrine. Compared to other opioids, tramadol has a lower addiction risk and a better overall safety profile, even though serious adverse effects of seizure and serotonin syndrome have been known to occur. Metabolism occurs in the liver by the cytochrome P450 system (CYP2B6, CYP2D6, CYP2C19 ,CYP3A4). *O*-desmethyltramadol is the most significant metabolite, since it has 200 times more affinity for MOR than the parent compound [54].

4.14. Tapentadol

Tapentadol is a relatively new (2008) and the exact mechanism of action is unknown. Although clinical relevance is unclear, preclinical animal studies have shown that tapentadol is a MOR agonist and norepinephrine re-uptake inhibitor (NRI). Tapentadol is avialble both as an immediate release formulation for acute moderate to severe pain in adults and as an extended release formulation for the management of moderate to severe chronic pain in adults when a continuous, around-the-clock opioid analgesic is needed for an extended period of time.No active analgesic metabolites have yet been identified. Tapentadol is primarily metabolized by gluronidation , where 99% of the parent molecule and its metabolites are excreted by the kidney.

Tapentadol exhibits low plasma protein binding (~20%). Tapentadol does not induce or inhibit P450 enzymes. Thus clinically relevant interactions mediated by the cytochrome P450 system are unlikely to occur. No clinically significant findings have been found in drug-drug interactions with acetaminophen, aspirin, naproxen, probenecid, omeprazole, and metaclopramide. Adverse effects appear to be dose-related and include sleepiness, dry mouth, nausea, and vertigo [55].

4.15. Naloxone

Naloxone is a semi-synthetic MOR antagonist, related to the opiate thebaine. Naloxone is a competitive antagonist at mu, kappa, and delta opioid receptors, with its highest affinity at MOR. Naloxone has a rapid onset of action and can quickly reverse the effects of opioid agonists and thus its primary clinical use is for rapid reversal of opioid overdose. Naloxone has been formulated in combination with opioid agonists (e.g. buprenorphine) in an effort to reduce the potential for abuse [56].

4.16. Naltrexone

Naltrexone is a synthetic competitive anatagonist at mu, kappa, and delta opioid receptors. It is used primarily as an oral formulation for detoxifing opioid abusers and addicts but also as an extended release injection for opioid dependence [57]. However, naltrexone has also shown efficacy and has been approved for alcohol dependence [58]. Naltrexone is metabolised mainly to 6β-naltrexol, which is also a competitive anatagonist at opioid receptors, by the liver enzyme dihydrodiol dehydrogenase [57].

5. Adverse Effects

5.1. Common Adverse Effects of Opioids

Because they act at many of the same receptors, most of the commonly prescribed opioids share a similar overall side-effect profile, whether they are prescribed for acute or chronic pain conditions. Common dose-dependent adverse effects of opioids include constipation, nausea, vomiting, dizziness, sedation, dry skin, pruritus, mental clouding, impaired psychomotor function, myoclonus, urinary retention, and respiratory depression [16, 59]. The severity of each adverse effect varies among the opioids and can be limited by using lower starting doses, longer dose intervals, and/or slower titration. The formulation can also alter the adverse effect profile, particularly if metabolites contribute significantly to the adverse effect profile.

5.1.1. Constipation

Constipation is a common adverse effect of opioid administration and is often a major limiting factor to dose escalation [16]. Due to different definitions of constipation and reporting methods (e.g., patient vs physician criteria), estimates of prevalence vary over a broad range, generally between 41% and 95% [23, 60]. Tolerance usually does not develop to the constipation effect, so prophylaxis is normally the preferred option. Stool softening and/or bowl stimulating laxative agents may be used initially; however, stronger therapies may be needed. Another approach is the administration of opioid antagonists that do not readily pass the blood-brain barrier and thus block the peripheral opioid receptors in the gastrointestinal tract, but do not reverse the central nervous system analgesic effects. Examples are methylnaltrexone and alvimopan [61-63]

5.1.2. Nausea and Vomiting

Nausea and vomiting signals are initiated within the vomiting center located in the medulla. The center receives signals from the gastrointestinal tract, cerebral cortex, vestibular system, and the chemoreceptor zone. Opioids stimulate the chemoreceptor zone and thus promote nausea and vomiting [16]. The effect is even more common in ambulatory patients, because of the additive effect of vestibular stimulation. Symptoms can be attenuated by the use of anti-emetics such as prochlorperazine or scopolamine [64].

5.1.3. Mental Clouding

Opioids can cause sedation, drowsiness, confusion, dizziness, or unsteadiness [16]. These symptoms usually develop within the first few days of therapy and usually resolve in 3 to 5 days [65]. Reducing the dose can ameliorate the severity of many of these symptoms. Particular attention should be paid to this adverse effect when prescribing opioids to the elderly, since many of them are at risk of falling and sustaining further injury [66].

5.1.4. Myoclonus

Opioid-induced myoclonus (a brief, involuntary twitch or spasm of muscle) occurs mainly in the perioperative setting and in chronic opioid users [16]. The phenomenon is not well understood, but might involve the accumulation of opioid metabolites [67].

5.1.5. Urinary Retention

Opioids increase contractions of the ureter and tone of the urinary sphincter, and decrease the force produced by contraction of the detrusor muscle. This in turn decreases the attention to full bladder and can lead to urinary retention. This is a frequent side effect seen mostly in males and may persist 10 – 20 hours following single epidural or intrathecal opioid administration [38].

5.1.6. Pruritus

Patients receiving opioids can develop pruritus (the sensation relieved by itching) [68]. It is more common with intraspinal administration [69]. The sensation is usually localized to the face and torso regions. The mechanism appears to be centrally mediated, but it is not completely understood. Research has implicated a number of possible mediators, including histamine, prostaglandins, tachykinins (substance P), endogenous opioid peptides, serotonin, and interleukins. Control can be maintained with titrated doses of naloxone or nalbuphine [70].

5.1.7. Respiratory Depression

Respiratory depression is the major toxicity of the MOR agonists and is usually the cause of death from overdose [16]. Opioids directly affect the respiratory control centers located in the medulla, particularly the potine and bulbar brainstem regions. Respiratory rate and tidal volume initially decrease, causing a decrease in minute ventilation. In addition, the patient's body becomes less responsive to carbon dioxide tension that normally is monitored by the medullary respiratory centers. Development of respiratory depression occurs mainly because of an overdose. Reducing opioid dosage may alleviate mild respiratory depression; severe cases require the use of opioid receptor antagonists [71].

5.1.8. Cardiovascular System

Cardiovascular adverse effects are uncommon when therapeutic doses of opioids are administered. Some opioids, such as morphine, stimulate the release of histamine, thus leading to vasodilation and hypotension [72]. Other opioids, such as fentanyl, sufentanil, alfentanil, and remifentanil, do not release histamine. Methadone and d-propoxyphene have received attention for their ability to induce QTc prolongation and torsades de pointes [73, 74].

5.2. Other Effects

5.2.1. Opioid-induced Hyperalgesia

Opioid-induced hyperalgesia clinically manifests as an increased or enhanced pain response to noxious stimuli during opioid treatment [75]. It is different from the development of tolerance and is normally associated with long-term use and/or high doses of opioids [25]. The phenomenon is not at all well understood and the extent to which it occurs in humans is not known. Accumulation of opioid metabolites such as morphine-3-glucuronide, cell apoptosis of GABA (γ-amino butyric acid) neurons, and/or NMDA (*N*-methl D-aspartate) receptor agonism have all been suggested to be involved in promoting opioid-induced hyperalgesia in animal studies [76, 77].

5.2.2. Immunosuppression

Opioid effects on the immune system have been suspected for over a 100 years. Within the last decade, more than 600 publications describing opioid immunologic effects have been published. The effects vary depending on the opioid administered and the susceptibility of the patient. The effect might be related to opioid receptors located on immune cells or within the CNS and suppress the humoral immune response [78]. It is not clear if these changes are clinically significant for the healthy patient, but they might be for immunocompromised patients. It remains an area of ongoing study [79].

5.2.3. Hypogonadism

Hypogondalism occurs due to the disruption of the hypothalamic-pituitary-gonadal axis and the resultant changes in many key hormone levels. Opioid receptors are prevalent in the hypothalamus and thus gonadal function can be altered by opioid drugs [80]. In addition, direct effects on the pituitary and the testes have been documented [80, 81]. Opioid receptor activation results in a cascade effect, starting with the disruption of the secretion of gonadotrophin releasing hormone, which in turn affects luteinizing hormone and follicle stimulating hormone, in addition to changes in testosterone or estradial secretion from the gonads [82, 83]. Opioids have also been reported to reduce testosterone secretion by increasing prolactin levels. [84]Testosterone concentrations have been documented to decline greater than 50% within a few hours after taking an opioid and return to normal within 24-72 hours after cessation [85]. Opioid-induced hypogonadism can lead to erectile dysfunction, impotence, loss of muscle mass in men, and irregular periods or amenorrhea in women [86, 87]. Flushing, sweating, decreased libido, infertility, osteopenia, osteoporosis, and depression can occur in both sexes.

5.2.4. Tolerance

During the course of multiple-dose opioid therapy, patients often experience a reduction in the therapeutic effect (i.e., 'tolerance' develops) [25]. Compensation for this reduction in effect is simply met by administering higher doses of the drug. Tolerance develops rapidly for effects such as analgesia and respiratory depression, but much less rapidly for constipation and miosis (the latter being convenient for differential diagnosis of opioid overdose). Switching to other opioids under these conditions might not necessarily restore analgesia because of the development of cross-tolerance to drugs that work by the same mechanism. It is important to recognize that (i) tolerance develops to almost every drug, but is often not as clinically evident as it is for opioids, and (ii) it is an independent phenomenon from addiction and is not *prima facie* evidence of addiction [88].

5.2.5. Physical Dependence

Physical dependence is the body's physiological adaptation that develops in response to continuous exposure to a drug [89]. It is not observed directly, but is manifested by 'withdrawal signs' that occur following abrupt reduced exposure to the drug or administration of an antagonist [89]. The phenomena of physical dependence is not limited to opioids, but withdrawal signs are drug-class specific. Opioid withdrawal signs include yawning, lacrimation, sneezing, agitation, tremor, insomnia, fever, tachycardia, and other signs of hyperexcitability of the sympathetic nervous system. Physical dependence and tolerance are different phenomena [89]. Physical dependence develops to almost every drug and it is an independent phenomenon from addiction. Despite the similarity in terminology, physical dependence is not the same thing as psychological 'dependence' on a drug and is not *prima facie* evidence of addiction.

5.2.6. Abuse/Misuse/Addiction

Like most other substances that produce biological effects, opioids are misused, abused, and pose the potential for addiction. Addiction is a complex interplay of biological, psychological, and environmental factors that is beyond the scope of the present coverage. The interested reader is directed to the many comprehensive and authoritative reviews [90-92].

6. Summary and Conclusions

Opioids are the mainstay of treatment for moderate to severe pain in both the acute and chronic pain settings. All opioids are not created equal and variability in both the pharmacokinetics and pharmacodynamics of many opioids makes prescribing these analgesics slightly difficult. In addition, the analgesic properties of opioids are normally limited by the incidence and severity of adverse effects. Therefore, it becomes imperative that a prescriber posses the current knowledge of opioid pharmacology and apply a patient specific, patient focused approach that will not only address a patient's pain etiology but minimize and reduce potential adverse effects.

REFERENCES

[1] Brownstein MJ. A brief history of opiates, opioid peptides, and opioid receptors. *Proc Natl Acad Sci* U S A. 1993 Jun 15;90(12):5391-3.

[2] Scarborough J, Porter R, Teich M. *The opium poppy in Hellenistic and Roman medicine Drugs and Narcotics in History:* Cambridge University Press; 1995.

[3] Huxtable RJ, Schwarz SKW. *The Isolation of Morphine—First Principles in Science and Ethics. Molecular Interventions.* 2001 October 1, 2001;1(4):189-91.

[4] Fine PG, Portenoy RK. *A Clinical Guide to Opioid Analgesia. Minneapolis:* Healthcare Information Programs; 2004.

[5] Thorpe DH. Opiate structure and activity--a guide to understanding the receptor. *Anesth Analg.* 1984 Feb;63(2):143-51.

[6] Goldstein A. Opioid peptides endorphins in pituitary and brain. *Science.* 1976 Sep 17;193(4258):1081-6.

[7] Koneru A, Satyanarayana S, Rizwan S. Endogenous Opioids: Their Physiological Role and Receptors. *Global Journal of Pharmacology.* 2009;3(3):149-53.

[8] Akil H, Watson SJ, Young E, Lewis ME, Khachaturian H, Walker JM. Endogenous opioids: biology and function. *Annu Rev Neurosci.* 1984;7:223-55.

[9] Waldhoer M, Bartlett SE, Whistler JL. Opioid receptors. *Annu Rev Biochem.* 2004;73:953-90.

[10] Trescot AM, Datta S, Lee M, Hansen H. Opioid pharmacology. *Pain Physician.* 2008 Mar;11(2 Suppl):S133-53.

[11] Meng F, Xie GX, Thompson RC, Mansour A, Goldstein A, Watson SJ, et al. Cloning and pharmacological characterization of a rat kappa opioid receptor. *Proc Natl Acad Sci* U S A. 1993 Nov 1;90(21):9954-8.

[12] Holzer P. Opioid receptors in the gastrointestinal tract. *Regul Pept.* 2009 Jun 5;155(1-3):11-7.

[13] Jordan B, Devi LA. Molecular mechanisms of opioid receptor signal transduction. *British Journal of Anaesthesia.* 1998;81:12-9.

[14] Vallejo R, Barkin RL, Wang VC. Pharmacology of Opioids in the Treatment of Chronic Pain Syndromes. *Pain Physician.* 2011;14:E343-E60.

[15] Choi YS, Billings JA. Opioid antagonists: a review of their role in palliative care, focusing on use in opioid-related constipation. *J Pain Symptom Manage.* 2002 Jul;24(1):71-90.

[16] McNicol E. Opioid Analgesics: Administration Issues, Side-effect management, and equianalgesic conversion. *Adv Stud Pharm.* 2008;5(1):16-25.

[17] Stevens RA, Ghazi SM. *Routes of Opioid Analgesic Therapy in the Management of Cancer Pain. Cancer Control.* 2000;7(2):132-41.

[18] Oldendorf WH, Hyman S, Braun L, Oldendorf SZ. Blood-brain barrier: penetration of morphine, codeine, heroin, and methadone after carotid injection. *Science.* 1972 Dec 1;178(64):984-6.

[19] Smith HS. Opioid metabolism. *Mayo Clin Proc.* 2009 Jul;84(7):613-24.

[20] Johnson SJ. Opioid Safety in Patients With Renal or Hepatic Dysfunction. *Pain Treatment Topics.* 2007:1-9.

[21] Hudcova J, McNicol E, Quah C, Lau J, Carr DB. Patient controlled opioid analgesia versus conventional opioid analgesia for postoperative pain. *Cochrane Database Syst Rev.* 2006(4):CD003348.
[22] Colson J, Koyyalagunta D, Falco FJ, Manchikanti L. A systematic review of observational studies on the effectiveness of opioid therapy for cancer pain. *Pain Physician.* 2011 Mar-Apr;14(2):E85-102.
[23] Kalso E, Edwards JE, Moore RA, McQuay HJ. Opioids in chronic non-cancer pain: systematic review of efficacy and safety. *Pain.* 2004 Dec;112(3):372-80.
[24] Eisenberg E, McNicol E, Carr DB. Opioids for neuropathic pain. *Cochrane Database Syst Rev.* 2006;3:CD006146.
[25] Ballanty JC, Shin NS. Efficacy of Opioids for Chronic Pain: A Review of the Evidence. *Clin J Pain.* 2008;24(6):469-78.
[26] Heinke B, Gingl E, Sandkuhler J. Multiple targets of mu-opioid receptor-mediated presynaptic inhibition at primary afferent Adelta- and C-fibers. *J Neurosci.* 2011 Jan 26;31(4):1313-22.
[27] Gibson PG, Ryan NM. Cough pharmacotherapy: current and future status. *Expert Opin Pharmacother.* 2011 Aug;12(11):1745-55.
[28] Wee B. Chronic cough. *Curr Opin Support Palliat Care.* 2008 Jun;2(2):105-9.
[29] McNeil-PPC Inc. LOPERAMIDE and LOPERAMIDE-SIMETHICONE Professional Product Information. 2011.
[30] Hain RD, Miser A, Devins M, Wallace WH. Strong opioids in pediatric palliative medicine. *Paediatr Drugs.* 2005;7(1):1-9.
[31] Anderson BJ, Palmer GM. Recent developments in the pharmacological management of pain in children. *Curr Opin Anaesthesiol.* 2006 Jun;19(3):285-92.
[32] Zernikow B, Lindena G. Long-acting morphine for pain control in paediatric oncology. *Med Pediatr Oncol.* 2001 Apr;36(4):451-8.
[33] Himelstein BP. Palliative care for infants, children, adolescents, and their families. *J Palliat Med.* 2006 Feb;9(1):163-81.
[34] Drake R, Longworth J, Collins JJ. Opioid rotation in children with cancer. *J Palliat Med.* 2004 Jun;7(3):419-22.
[35] Pergolizzi J, Boger RH, Budd K, Dahan A, Erdine S, Hans G, et al. Opioids and the management of chronic severe pain in the elderly: consensus statement of an International Expert Panel with focus on the six clinically most often used World Health Organization Step III opioids (buprenorphine, fentanyl, hydromorphone, methadone, morphine, oxycodone). *Pain Pract.* 2008 Jul-Aug;8(4):287-313.
[36] Actavis Kadian LLC. KADIAN® (morphine sulfate extended-release) Capsules Prescribing Information. 2010.
[37] APP Pharmaceuticals. *Astramorph (Morphine Sulfate Injection, USP) Preservative Free Prescribing Insert.* June 2008.
[38] Baxter. *Duramorph (morphine sulfate injection) prescribing information.* 2011.
[39] King Pharmaceuticals. *AVINZA (morphine sulfate extended-release capsules) prescribing information.* 2011.
[40] Purdue Pharmaceuticals. *MS Contin (morphine sulfate controlled-release) Tablets Prescribing Information.* 2011.
[41] Xanodyne Pharmaceuticals. Oramorph SR (morphine sulfate) sustained release tablets prescribing information. 2011.

[42] Armstrong S, Cozza K. Pharmacokinetic drug interactions of morphine, codeine, and their derivatives: Theory and clinical reality. . *Psychosomatics*. 2003;44:515-20.

[43] Picara. *Duragesic (Fentanyl Transdermal System)*. 2009.

[44] Abbott Laboratories. VICODIN ES® *(hydrocodone bitartrate and acetaminophen tablets, USP)*. 2011.

[45] Abbott Laboratories. *Vicoprofen (hydrocodone bitartrate and ibuprofen tablets)*. 2009.

[46] Purdue Pharma. *Dilaudid (hydromorphone hydrochloride)*. 2009.

[47] Purdue Pharma. *Oxycontin (Oxycodone HCl Controlled Release) Tablets*. 2010.

[48] Endo Pharmaceuticals. *OPANA ER (oxymorphone hydrochloride) Extended-Release tablets*, CII. 2010.

[49] Pergolizzi J, Aloisi AM, Dahan A, Filitz J, Langford R, Likar R, et al. Current knowledge of buprenorphine and its unique pharmacological profile. *Pain Pract*. 2010 Sep-Oct;10(5):428-50.

[50] Purdue Pharma. *Butrans (buprenorphine) Transdermal System*, CIII. 2010.

[51] Sanofi Aventis. *Demerol (meperidine hydrocholoride, USP)*. 2011.

[52] Lynch M. A review of the use of methadone for the treatment of chronic noncancer pain. *Pain Res Manage* 2005;10:133-44.

[53] Krantz M, Lewkowiez L, Hays H, Woodroffe M, Robertson A, Mehler P. Torsade de pointes associated with very high dose methadone. *Ann Intern Med*. 2002;137:501-4.

[54] PriCara. ULTRAM ER (tramadol HCI) *Extended-Release Tablets*. 2009.

[55] PriCara. NUCYNTA® (*tapentadol) Tablets*. 2010.

[56] Reckitt Benckiser Pharmaceuticals Inc. *Suboxone (buprenorphine and naloxone) prescribing information*. 2010.

[57] Alkermes. *Vivitrol (naltrexone for extended release injectable suspension) prescribing information*. 2010.

[58] Garbutt JC. Efficacy and tolerability of naltrexone in the management of alcohol dependence. *Curr Pharm Des*. 2010;16(19):2091-7.

[59] McNicol E, Horowicz-Mehler N, Fisk RA, Bennett K, Gialeli-Goudas M, Chew PW, et al. Management of opioid side effects in cancer-related and chronic noncancer pain: a systematic review. *J Pain*. 2003 Jun;4(5):231-56.

[60] Robinson CB, Fritch M, Hullett L, Petersen MA, Sikkema S, Theuninck L, et al. Development of a protocol to prevent opioid-induced constipation in patients with cancer: a research utilization project. *Clin J Oncol Nurs*. 2000 Mar-Apr;4(2):79-84.

[61] Kurz A, Sessler DI. Opioid-induced bowel dysfunction: pathophysiology and potential new therapies. *Drugs*. 2003;63(7):649-71.

[62] Schmidt WK. Alvimopan* (ADL 8-2698) is a novel peripheral opioid antagonist. *Am J Surg*. 2001 Nov;182(5A Suppl):27S-38S.

[63] Foss JF. A review of the potential role of methylnaltrexone in opioid bowel dysfunction. *Am J Surg*. 2001 Nov;182(5A Suppl):19S-26S.

[64] Porreca F, Ossipov MH. Nausea and vomiting side effects with opioid analgesics during treatment of chronic pain: mechanisms, implications, and management options. *Pain Med*. 2009 May-Jun;10(4):654-62.

[65] Mercadante S, Portenoy RK. Opioid poorly-responsive cancer pain. Part 1: clinical considerations. *J Pain Symptom Manage*. 2001 Feb;21(2):144-50.

[66] Saunders KW, Dunn KM, Merrill JO, Sullivan M, Weisner C, Braden JB, et al. Relationship of opioid use and dosage levels to fractures in older chronic pain patients. *J Gen Intern Med.* 2010 Apr;25(4):310-5.
[67] Mercadante S. Pathophysiology and treatment of opioid-related myoclonus in cancer patients. *Pain.* 1998 Jan;74(1):5-9.
[68] Reich A, Szepietowski JC. Opioid-induced pruritus: an update. *Clin Exp Dermatol.* 2010 Jan;35(1):2-6.
[69] Chaney MA. Side effects of intrathecal and epidural opioids. *Can J Anaesth.* 1995 Oct;42(10):891-903.
[70] Miller JL, Hagemann TM. Use of pure opioid antagonists for management of opioid-induced pruritus. *American Journal of Health-System Pharmacy.* 2011 August 1, 2011;68(15):1419-25.
[71] Dahan A, Aarts L, Smith TW. Incidence, Reversal, and Prevention of Opioid-induced Respiratory Depression. *Anesthesiology.* 2010 Jan;112(1):226-38.
[72] Brunton L, Lazo J, Parker K. Goodman and Gilman's *The Pharmacologica Basis of Therapeutics,* 11th Edition. New York: McGraw-Hill; 2006.
[73] Krantz M, Mehler P. Synthetic opioids and QT prolongation. *Arch Intern Med.* 2003;163:1615.
[74] Walker P, Klein D, Kasza L. High dose methadone and ventricular arrhythmias: A report of three cases. *Pain.* 2003;103:321-4.
[75] Lee M, Silverman SM, Hansen H, Patel VB, Manchikanti L. A comprehensive review of opioid-induced hyperalgesia. *Pain Physician.* 2011 Mar-Apr;14(2):145-61.
[76] Mercadante S, Ferrera P, Villari P, Arcuri E. Hyperalgesia: An emerging iatrogenpression ic syndrome. *J Pain Symptom Manage.* 2003;26:769-75.
[77] Mao J, Sung B, Ji R, Lim G. Neuronal apoptosis associated with morphine tolerance: Evidence for an opioid-induced neurotoxic mechanism. *J Neurosci.* 2002;22:7650-61.
[78] Budd K. Pain management: is opioid immunosuppression a clinical problem? *Biomedicine & Pharmacotherapy.* 2006;60:310-7.
[79] Sacerdote P. Opioid-induced immunosuppression. *Curr Opin Support Palliat Care.* 2008 Mar;2(1):14-8.
[80] Vuong C, Van Uum S, O'Dell L, Lutfy K, Friedman T. The effects of opioids and opioid analogs on animal and human endocrine systems. *Endocr Rev.* 2010;31:98-132.
[81] Adams M, Sewing B, Forman J, Meyer E, Cicero T. Opioid-induced suppression of rat testicular function. *J Pharmacol Exp Ther.* 1993;266:323-8.
[82] Azizi F, Vagenakis A, Longcope C, Ingbar S, Braverman L. Decreased serum testosterone concentration in male heroin and methadone addicts. *Steroids.* 1973;22:467-72.
[83] Mehmanesh H, Almeida O, Nikolarakis K, Herz A. Hypothalamic LH-RH release after acute and chronic treatment with morphine studied in a combined in vivo/in vitro model. *Brain Research.* 1988;451:69-76.
[84] Delitala G, Grossman A, Besser G. The participation of hypothalamic dopamine in morphine-induced prolactin release in man. *Clin Endocrinol.* 1983;19:437-44.
[85] Bliesener N, Albrecht S, Schwager A, Weckbecker K, Lichtermann D, Klingmuller D. Plasma testosterone and sexual function in men receiving buprenorphine maintenance for opioid dependence. *J Clin Endocrinol Metab.* 2005;90:203-6.

[86] Reddy RG, Aung T, Karavitaki N, Wass JA. Opioid induced hypogonadism. *BMJ.* 2010;341:c4462.
[87] Hallinan R, Byrne A, Agho K, McMahon C, Tynan P, Attia J. Erectile dysfunction in men receiving methadone and buprenorphine maintenance treatment. *J Sex Med.* 2008;5:684-92.
[88] Benyamin R, Trescot AM, Datta S, Buenaventura R, Adlaka R, Sehgal N, et al. Opioid complications and side effects. *Pain Physician.* 2008 Mar;11(2 Suppl):S105-20.
[89] Kosten TR, George TP. The neurobiology of opioid dependence: implications for treatment. *Sci Pract Perspect.* 2002 Jul;1(1):13-20.
[90] Amato L, Davoli M, Vecchi S, Ali R, Farrell M, Faggiano F, et al. Cochrane systematic reviews in the field of addiction: what's there and what should be. *Drug Alcohol Depend.* 2011 Jan 15;113(2-3):96-103.
[91] Raffa RB, Pergolizzi JV, Jr. Opioid formulations designed to resist/deter abuse. *Drugs.* 2010 Sep 10;70(13):1657-75.
[92] Strassels SA. Economic burden of prescription opioid misuse and abuse. *J Manag Care Pharm.* 2009 Sep;15(7):556-62.

In: Opioids: Pharmacology, Clinical Uses and Adverse Effects ISBN 978-1-61942-101-1
Editors: Djavakhi Tvildiani and Kakha Gegechkori

Chapter 6

NEWLY DEVELOPED STRONG OPIOIDS: PRESENT AND FUTURE ASPECTS

Sang Ryong Jeon and Jin Hoon Park
Department of Neurological Surgery, Asan Medical Center, University of Ulsan College of Medicine, Seoul, Korea

ABSTRACT

Strong opioids are widely used for several types of pain, such as acute or chronic, and moderate to severe pain. However, there have been many reports which describe its side effects, such as nausea, vomiting, constipation, analgesia, addiction, etc. Therefore, efforts to overcome these side effects and increase their effectiveness are made. Specific mechanisms of several opioids which are newly developed are described here and future aspects of strategy for developing strong opioids are explained.

For example, hydromorphone has a strong analgesic effect, but because of its short acting duration and fluctuation of blood concentration, there is a possibility of addiction. Also, it is inappropriate for basal pain. Prolonged releasing hydromorphone is developed by osmotic-controlled release technology (Jurnista®), and this can be used basal pain as well as breakthrough pain. In addition, delayed gastrointestinal(GI) mobility with the use of opiods has been well known. Naloxone, which was added to oxycodone, acts as an antagonist of receptors in the GI system and can improve constipation symptoms, developed under the name of Targin®. Furthermore, new opioids are being developed to have synergistic analgesic action between the receptor and other pain related receptors such as a-adrenergic (Tapentadol®). Through these newly developing opioids, we can consider future aspects of opiods as well as concepts for medical pain therapy.

INTRODUCTION

Opioids, which vary in type and pharmacokinetics, are frequently used to manage pain[56, 85, 106]. Strong opioids, such as morphine, hydromorphone and oxycodone, are widely used for several types of pain, including acute and chronic, moderate-to-severe cancer pain as well as non-cancer pain[9, 26, 36, 43, 47, 48, 60-62, 81, 97, 113, 117]. Such opioids, however, frequently have side effects, including nausea, vomiting, constipation, dizziness, sleepiness, and addiction[4, 6-8, 21, 22, 24, 34, 57, 58, 65, 70]. Different opioid formulations and delivery devices, with decreased side effects and increased effectiveness, have therefore been developed. Here we describe the mechanisms of action of three newly developed opioids and an intrathecal morphine pump, and we discuss future strategies for the development of strong opioids.

COMBINATION OF OXYCODONE AND NALOXONE

Oxycodone (6-deoxy-7, 8-dehydro-14-hydroxy-3-O-methyl-6-oxomorphine) is a semi-synthetic opioid analgesic, first derived from thebaine in 1916 and used since 1917 [25].Oxycodone binds to μ- κ-, and opioid receptors. Due to reduced first-pass hepatic clearance, the oral bioavailability of oxycodone (60–87%) is higher than that of morphine (about 20–30%) [83, 92].Controlled-release oxycodone (CRO) and immediate-release oxycodone (IRO) oral formulations have been developed. The CRO formulation uses a dual control matrix system and acts in two absorption phases, thus endowing it with biphasic analgesic effects. In the rapid initial absorption phase, 38% of the available dose is administered via a process with an absorption half-life ($T_{1/2}$) of 37 min. In the slow absorption phase, by contrast, the remaining 62% of the available dose is administered via a process with an absorption $T_{1/2}$ of 6.2 hours. These features of CRO permit analgesic effects with a rapid onset that last for 12 hours [18, 73]. In comparison, the IRO formulation induces pain relief as early as 15 minutes after administration and lasts for 4 hours [84]. Oxycodone is one of the most widely used opium analogs and numerous clinical studies have shown its analgesic efficacy in treating cancer and non-cancer chronic pain. [47, 86, 87, 104]. The immediate- and controlled-release formulations of oxycodone are equally effective and safe [45, 89, 101].

However, like all opioids, oxycodone is associated with adverse events including nausea, vomiting, and symptoms related to bowel dysfunction. These adverse events become obstacles to treatment with opioids, despite the clinical benefits of such drugs [25].Opioid-induced gastrointestinal (GI) side effects are caused by binding to opioid receptors in the GI tract, which causes reduced motility and secretion. Opioid-induced constipation (OIC) is the most common and troublesome GI side effect because it is persistent and not alleviated by tolerance. OIC affects 15–90% of patients and can reduce the analgesic efficacy of opioids by up to 30% [51, 74]. OIC may be managed prophylactically by co-administration of an opioid and an opioid antagonist.

One newly developed strong opioid agent consists of a combination of oxycodone PR (prolonged release) with oral naloxone PR in a 2:1 ratio (ONC) (Targin®, Mundipharma International Limited, Cambridge, UK). These opium analogs combine with receptors in the central nervous system (CNS) and peripheral nervous system (PNS), such as μ- and κ-opioid receptors. The clinical efficacy and pharmacokinetics of individually administered oxycodone PR and oral naloxone PR have been described.[14, 35, 52, 86] Naloxone is an opioid antagonist that has been used intravenously to treat opioid overdoses [83]. Intravenous naloxone has been shown to reverse all PNS- and CNS-mediated opioid effects by crossing the blood–brain barrier. However, when given orally, naloxone is extensively eliminated by hepatic first-pass metabolism, resulting in negligible systemic bioavailability (less than 2%)

[92]. Therefore, oral naloxone antagonizes the binding of oxycodone to opioid receptors in the GI tract but does not affect the analgesic efficacy of oxycodone [73, 92].

The optimal oxycodone:naloxone ratio in ONC was shown to be 2:1, with this formulation being bioequivalent to oxycodone PR in its analgesic efficacy. Moreover, this formulation has been shown to prevent OIC. Figure 1 shows the change in bowel function over time during follow up in ONC treated and oxycodone PR treated patients. It is clear that bowel function is superior in the former group. Naloxone had no impact on the analgesic effect of oxycodone when administered in ONCtablets [63, 99, 112]. By improving OIC, ONC has several clinical advantages for pain management. The dose ranges and comparatively short time to reach steady state may have benefits for initiation and titration [25], and the combination of an opioid agonist and antagonist in ONC may reduce the likelihood of opioid abuse [18, 84, 86]. The metabolism of the oxycodone/naloxone combination is the same as that of oxycodone; however, in patients with hepatic or renal impairments, naloxone may not be fully metabolized, thus affecting the analgesic effect of oxycodone. Therefore, as with most drugs, this formulation should be used with caution in patients with mild hepatic dysfunction and/or renal dysfunction and is contraindicated in patients with moderate-to-severe hepatic impairment[25, 45, 89, 101].

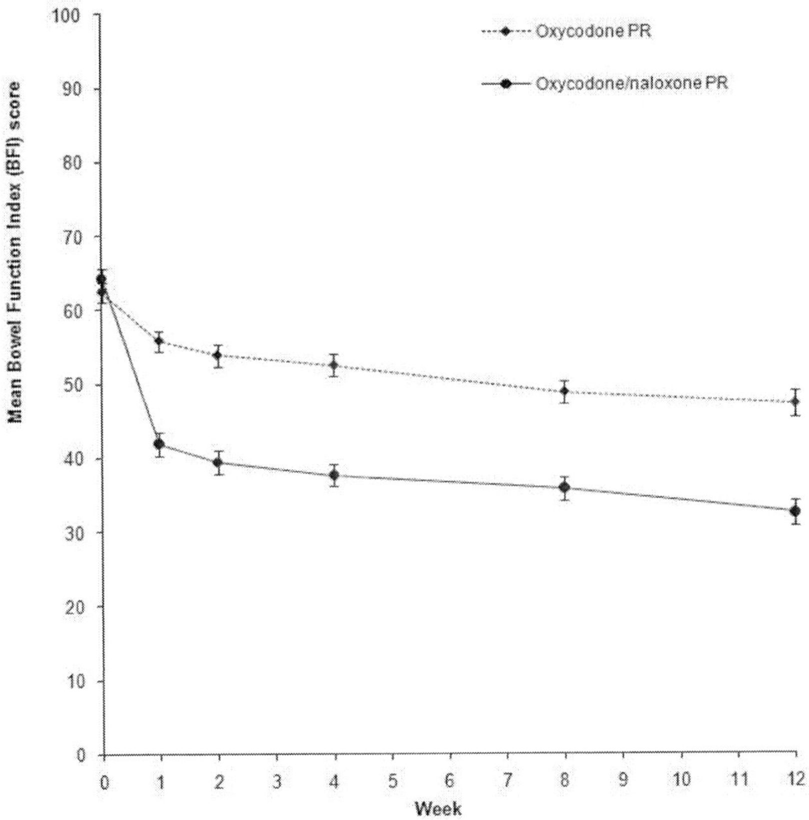

Figure 1. Mean Bowel Function Index score over time(Full analysis population : last observation carried forward analysis) (Figure reproduced from BMC Clinical Pharmacology 2010, 10:12 and adapted with permission of the authors; original figure published by BioMed Central).

Targin® has been approved for clinical use in Austria, Australia, Belgium, Canada, Cyprus, Denmark, Finland, Germany, Israel, Italy, Korea, Luxembourg, the Netherlands, Norway, Poland, the Republic of Ireland, the Slovak Republic, Sweden, Switzerland, and the United Kingdom[59]. Drugs under development for improved OIC management are also described below in the section on future strategies for the development of strong opioids.

SLOW-RELEASE HYDROMORPHONE

Hydromorphone has strong analgesic effects in patients suffering from severe pain, but its duration of action is short, requiring dosing several times per day and making it difficult to control variations in blood concentration [12, 81, 103]. Many studies have described its pharmacokinetics, with the view of developing a longer-acting drug [11, 13, 95, 107]. Hydromorphone is a morphine-like opioid agonist with a 5- to 7-fold greater potency than morphine and has been used to treat acute and chronic pain for almost 80 years [67]. Like morphine, its effects are primarily mediated by binding to μ-opioid receptors [90]. Hydromorphone also interacts with δ-opioid receptors, but to a lesser extent. Its pharmacologic profile is similar to that of morphine, but it has been associated with lower rates of pruritus, nausea, vomiting, sedation, and cognitive impairment [90]. As with morphine, there is no intrinsic limit to the analgesiceffects of hydromorphone, and adequate doses will relieve even the most severe pain. Orally administered hydromorphone is more potent than a number of other commonly used opioid agonists. The estimated equianalgesic doses are shown in Table 1 [12, 90].

OROS® hydromorphone (*Jurnista*™, Janssen Pharmaceutica N.V., Beerse, Belgium), which has slow-release pharmacokinetics, was developed to overcome the short duration of action of hydromorphone. OROS stands for osmotic-controlled release oral delivery system, resulting in consistent, long-lasting levels of analgesia [3, 23].The need for multiple daily doses of oral opioids has been associated with inconvenience for subjects and poor adherence to therapy, resulting in inadequate analgesia and diminished quality of life [27]. Furthermore, short-acting strong opioids have a higher addiction rate than longer-acting opioids [91]. Three opioids are currently available as oral, long-acting formulations: slow-release (SR) morphine sulfate, SR oxycodone, and OROS® hydromorphone. SR morphine sulfate and SR oxycodone require dosing at least twice daily, whereas OROS® hydromorphone can provide 24-hour analgesia with limited breakthrough pain [105].OROS® hydromorphone was shown to control moderate-to-severe basal pain, which could not be controlled with conventional hydromorphone due to the risk of addiction [5, 15, 28, 32, 66, 103].

Table 1. Ratios for conversion of select opioids tohydromorphone (oral administration)

Opioid	Conversion Ratio (Oral Opioid [mg]to Oral Hydromorphone [mg])
Morphine	5–7.5:1
Oxycodone	4:1
Codeine	27:1
Meperidine	40:1

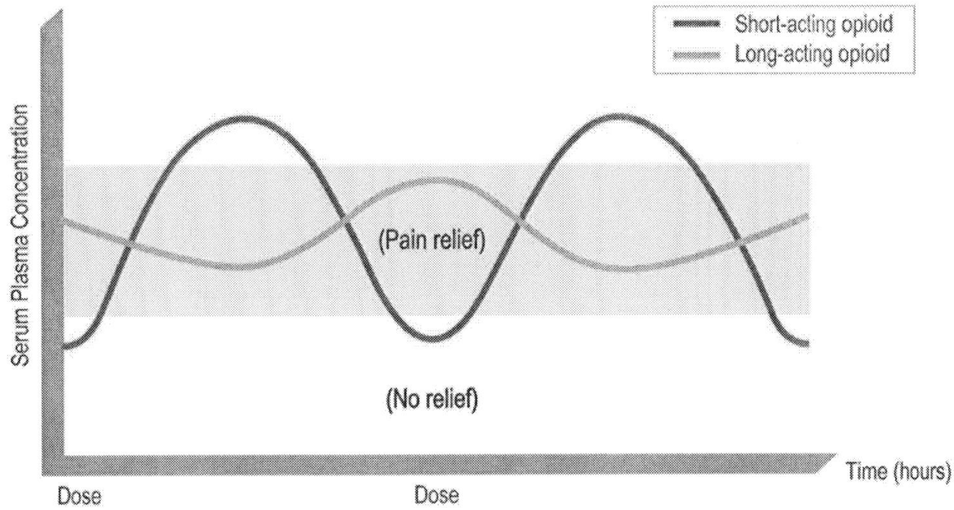

Figure 2. Long-acting opioids provide minimal fluctuation in plasma concentrations over extended periods of time.

Compared with immediate-release (IR) hydromorphone, OROS® hydromorphone provides more consistent drug delivery, with lower peak concentrations and reduced variability in plasma concentrations over time (Figure 2) [23]. Peak plasma concentrations of hydromorphone are achieved approximately 12 to 16 hours after administration of OROS® hydromorphone (Jurnista™), with 50% of peak levels attained within approximately 5 to 6 hours [3]. Steady-state concentrations are achieved after 2 days, at which time fluctuations in plasma level are reduced when compared with IR hydromorphone [17]. The OROS® delivery system enables approximately 80% of the total hydromorphone dose to be released in the colon. In contrast, administration of the IR formulations results in release of most of the drug in the upper GI tract. Hydromorphone is extensively metabolized in the liver and excreted in the urine. As with other strong opioids, hydromorphone can accumulate in the presence of renal failure and contribute to the development of side effects such as respiratory depression [67]. The adverse effects most frequently reported by patients receiving OROS® hydromorphone involve the GI and central nervous systems (Table 2)[90].

Table 3. Physical and Pharmacokinetic Characteristics of the Transdermal Fentanyl Device

Transdermal Device Strength (µg/h)	Transdermal Device Surface Area (cm^2)	Fentanyl Content (mg)	Mean(SD) Time to Maximal Concentration (h)	Mean(SD) Maxima Plasma Concentration (ng/mL)
12.5	5	1.25	27.5 (9.6)	0.3 (0.2)
25	10	2.5	38.1 (18.0)	0.6 (0.3)
50	20	5	34.8 (15.4)	1.4 (0.5)
75	30	7.5	33.5 (14.5)	1.7 (0.7)
100	40	10	36.8 (15.7)	2.5 (1.2)

Table 2. Adverse events occurring in ≥5% of patients withchronic pain treated with OROS® hydromorphone (N=570)

Event	Incidence, %
Nausea	25.3
Vomiting	21.6
Constipation	18.6
Somnolence	17.2
Headache	17.0
Dizziness	14.4
Diarrhea	11.1
Fatigue	8.9
Pruritus	8.4
Sweating, increased	8.2
Insomnia	7.9
Edema, lower limb	7.7
Anorexia	7.7
Influenza	7.5
Accident	7.5
Constipation, aggravated	7.2
Upper respiratory tract infection	6.7
Weakness	6.3
Pain, abdominal	5.6
Dry mouth	5.4
Dyspepsia	5.3
Anxiety	5.3
Dyspnea	5.3

Fentanyl Transdermal Patch

Fentanyl was introduced in 1960 to replace morphine and other opioids for use in cardiac surgery due to its greater potency (approximately 75- to 100-fold greater than that of morphine) [102]. Fentanyl can be delivered by intravenous (IV), transmucosal, buccal, epidural, intrathecal, and inhalational routes [69, 77, 78]. However, for practical and pharmacokinetic reasons, transdermal fentanyl is indicated only for the treatment of chronic pain, and can even be used in an outpatient setting. Transdermal fentanyl allows opioid analgesia to be provided in a discrete, convenient, noninvasive, and generally safe manner [41, 96, 98].

The transdermal patch system (Durogesic D-TRANS®,Janssen Pharmaceutica N.V., Beerse, Belgium) for delivering fentanyl causes the drug to be absorbed systemically by sustained dissolution over 72 h. While oral SR morphine, the standard opioid for chronic pain, has been associated with severe constipation and reduced patient quality of life [44, 76], a percutaneous transdermal fentanyl has been associated with lower rates of constipation and sedative actions [1, 79].Fentanyl has shown analgesic effects on neuropathic pain not susceptible to other general opioids [19, 76]. Fentanyl has many of the physicochemical properties essential for transdermal use [55]. Its high lipophilicity results in rapid diffusion into the lipophilic epidermal tissue with subsequent slow movement into the water-rich dermal tissue (Figure 3) [68]. This results in the formation of a depot in the keratinaceous layer of the epidermis. This depot formation accounts for the slow onset and prolonged effects of transdermally delivered fentanyl. Sites of application should be changed periodically to prevent serum concentration fluctuations resulting from the development of large depots resulting from consecutive use of the same site. Variations in skin thickness and degree of keratinization can alter the systemic bioavailability of fentanyl and account for much of the interindividual variability observed with transdermal fentanyl absorption [31, 46, 100]. A >50% difference in fentanyl permeability has been observed in different skin samples [54].

Although fentanyl can be detected in the serum within 1–2 hours of application of a transdermal patch, therapeutic serum concentrations require approximately 12–16 hours [30, 42, 88, 111]. The mean time to maximal serum concentration is about 36 hours, regardless of the release kinetics of the transdermal patch, but there is substantial intersubject variability (17–48 hours) [30, 82]. The detailed pharmacokinetic characteristics of different dose patches are illustrated in Table 3. As a potent opioid analgesic in a concentrated transdermal device system, its dose should be prescribed carefully by medical doctors [68, 76].

Intrathecal Morphine Pump

Direct delivery of opioids into the cerebral spinal fluid (CSF) within the intrathecal space avoids crossing the blood–brain barrier and results in smaller doses with higher efficacy than administration via oral, intravenous, or epidural routes. Implantable pumps for the delivery of intrathecal morphine have been used since 1981 [72]. Administration of smaller doses may reduce the systemic side effects of morphine, and direct delivery to the site of action allows a more rapid and effective response with fewer adverse effects [16, 39, 40, 71].

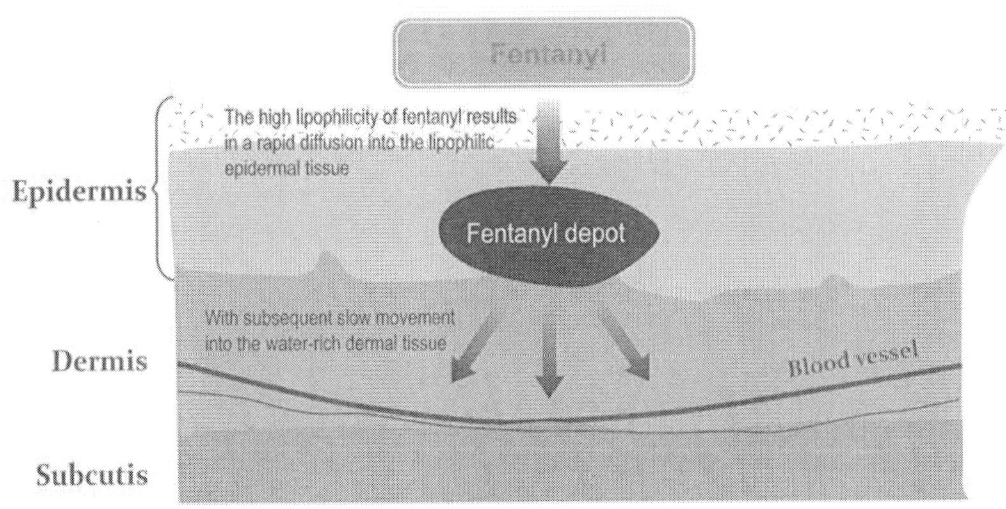

Figure 3. Cross-section of skin, showing that fentanyl, with high lipid solubility, readily enters the epidermal lipids and forms a depot at the dermal-epidermal junction. This depot slowly dissolves in the hydrophilic dermis and enters the cutaneous blood circulation.

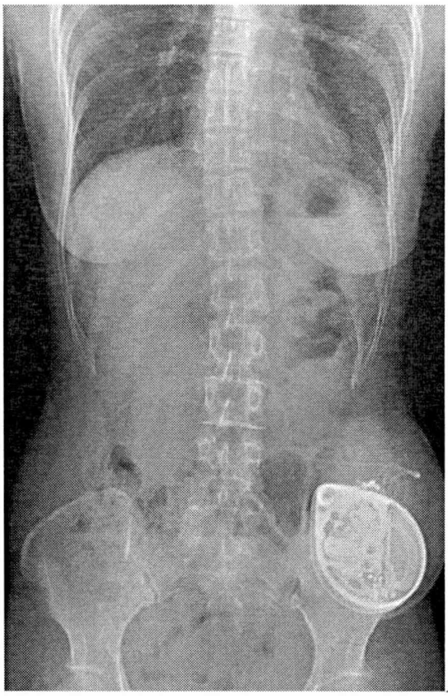

A

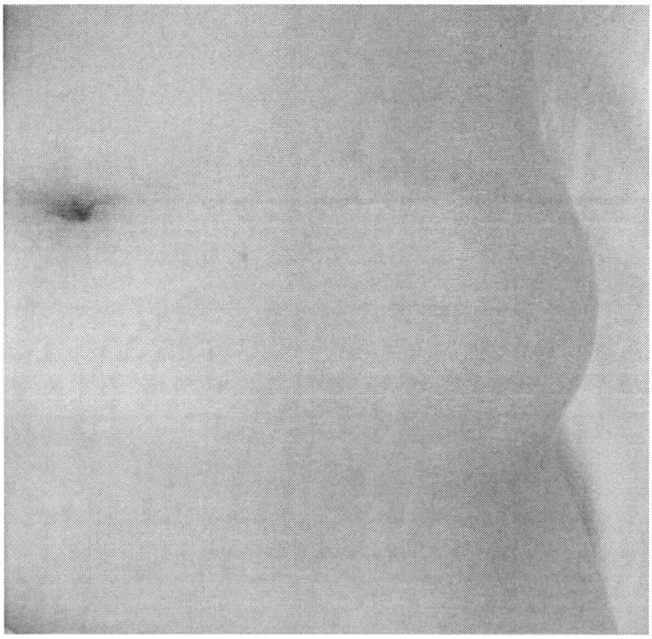

B

Figure 4. A 32-year-old female patient admitted with intractable post-traumatic pain after a traumatic accident. She suffered sustained back and bilateral leg pain, which was intractable to strongopioids except for continuous intravenous morphine injection.

A. Intrathecal implantation of a morphine pump. The catheter tip is located in the T8vertebral body level, with the pump in the left lower abdomen.

B. Photograph of the abdomen of the same patient, showing cyst-like swelling due to leakage of morphine around the pump.

Table 4. Conversion ratiosfor different methods of administration

Method of administration	Conversion Ratio
Oral : Intravenous dose	3:1
Intravenous : Epidural dose	10:1
Epidural : Intrathecal dose	10:1
Oral : Intrathecal dose	300:1

Morphine interacts predominantly with the μ-receptors on neurons. These μ-binding sites are discretely distributed throughout the human brain, with high densities in the posterior amygdala, hypothalamus, thalamus, caudate nucleus, putamen, and certain cortical areas. These binding sites are also found on the terminal axons of primary afferents within laminae I and II (substantia gelatinosa) of the spinal cord and in the spinal nucleus of the trigeminal nerve [29, 53, 114-116]. Morphine, with high hydrophilicity, penetrates the spinal cord slowly, allowing a considerable amount of the drug to ascend the cephalad in the CSF [10]. The mechanism of cephalad migration of morphine is thought to be due to bulk flow of the CSF [20], which ascends from the lumbar region, reaches the cisterna magna within 1–2 hours and reaches the fourth and lateral ventricles by 3-6 hours [20]. Morphine is predominantly metabolized in the liver, with its metabolism involving its conjugation with glucuronic acid to form the biologically inactive products, morphine-3 and morphine-6 glucuronides. These conjugates are predominantly excreted through the kidneys, with about 10% in the feces. Morphine is also eliminated by the kidneys, with 2–12% being excreted unchanged in the urine [64]. Intrathecal delivery of morphine via an indwelling pump may be effective in about 60% of patients with chronic pain of non-malignant origin [40]. Because these pumps deliver morphine directly to the sites of therapeutic action, it results in better analgesia at low doses and with few side effects [16, 39, 40]. Commercial intrathecal pump devices are available in the form of Infumorph® (Medtronic, Minneapolis, TN, USA); its intrathecal insertion and pump implantation are illustrated in Figure 4-A.

Such pump devices are indicated for patients with cancer or non-malignant pain who experience inadequate pain relief and/or intolerable side effects from systemic opioid therapy [50]. Other selection criteria include a life expectancy greater than 3 months, a body size sufficient to accept the bulk and weight of the pump, no evidence of infection, a favorable response to trial opioid treatment, objective evidence of pathology, psychological clearance, and no untreated substance abuse [50]. Infusion for a trial may include single or multiple doses or continuous infusion [71, 80].

A conservative method of determining the target dose of intraspinal morphine in a newly implanted patient is to convert the patient's daily oral and/or systemic opioid dose to an intraspinal morphine equivalent dose. After the oral or IV morphine equivalent is established, this dose should be converted to an epidural or intrathecal morphine dose, as described in Table 4 [50]. The mean daily intrathecally injected dose of morphine was found to be 2.75 mg (range, 0.25–8 mg) [94].

Intrathecally administered morphine results in a slow onset and long duration of anti-nociception, but it has also been associated with certain side effects [10]. The pharmacological side effects of intrathecal morphine therapy, such as pruritus, nausea/vomiting, urinary retention, constipation, mental status change, and respiratory depression, can be easily antagonized by the μ-receptor antagonist naloxone [10]. The side effects of intrathecal morphine therapy are usually common during the initiation phase of treatment and generally resolve with standard medical management during the first 3 months [2].

Other possible disadvantages of intrathecal pumps compared with intravenous drug administration include higher costs, postoperative meningitis, catheter dislocation, malfunction, inconvenience refilling the device with morphine every 3 months, and leakage around the device (Figure 4-B). To minimize such risks, intrathecal opioid drug administration using implantable pumps should be decided on by interdisciplinary teams at specialized centers [49].

Table 5. New formulations to deter abuse

Current name	Active Drug	Type of Formulation	Manufacture
Remoxy™	Oxycodone (Extended Release)	Gelatin Capsule highly viscous liquid	Pain therapeutics King pharmaceuticals
COL-003	Oxycodone (Extended Release)	Mult-iparticulate matrix with particles in Waxy excipient base	Collegium Pharmaceutical Inc.
ELI-216	Oxycodone (Extended Release)	Capsule containing separate oxycodone and naltrexone pellets	ElitePharmaceuticals
Embeda®	Morphine (Extended Release)	Pellets of morphine surrounding an inner core of naltrexone	King Pharmaceuticals
TQ-1017	Tramadol (Extended Release)	Transforms into viscous substance in the presence of solvents	TheraQuest Bioscience
Acurox®	Oxycodone (Immediate Release)	Co-formulated with subtherapeutic doses of niacin	Acura Pharmaceuticals King Pharmaceuticals

FUTURE STRATEGIES FOR THE DEVELOPMENT OF STRONG OPIOIDS

There are two directions for the development of strong opioids. One is to develop new molecules that do not have side effects such as OIC and that have increased efficacy. Another direction is to create new formulations that are associated with lower rates of abuse or side effects. New formulations developed to reduce abuse are described in Table 5 [93].

Tapentadol ((-)-(1*R*,2*R*)-3-(3-dimethylamino-1-ethyl-2-methyl-propyl)-phenol hydrochloride) is a novel, centrally acting analgesic with two mechanisms of action, μ-opioid receptor (MOR) agonism and noradrenaline reuptake inhibition (NRI), in a single molecule [108-110]. In addition to the ability of both mechanisms of action to produce analgesia individually, they can also interact synergistically at the spinal and supraspinal levels. The NRI component can produce an 'opioid-sparing effect', such that a moderate MOR-agonistic activity is sufficient (in concert with the moderate NRI activity) to produce potent analgesia, thus reducing opioid-induced side effects. Indeed, despite having a 50-fold lower affinity for the MOR, tapentadol is only 2- to 3-fold less potent than morphine across a variety of preclinical pain models[109]. These findings clearly indicate that: a) the NRI component of tapentadol contributes to its analgesic effect; and b) it does so in a supraadditive/synergistic manner. Tapentadol has demonstrated potent analgesia in patients with acute and chronic pain, as well as having a substantially improved GI side-effect profile [33, 37, 38].Although it has been recommended for treatment [75], there are still unmet clinical needs in the management of OIC, an increasingly relevant problem arising from the extensive use of opioids for the relief of chronic pain, often associated with benign conditions.

Several new pharmacological approaches are being developed, including the assessment of improved motility and secretagogue agents that are effective in OIC. Other approaches are directed at the reversal of peripheral opiate effects in the gut while maintaining the desired analgesic efficacy. Although subcutaneous methylnaltrexone is already approved for induction of laxation in advanced illness, several new approaches are promising, including combinations of opioids with PR naloxone, NKTR-118, and TD-1211. An evidence-based management approach for OIC will be more feasible after the new generation of drugs is formally and thoroughly studied in large, high-quality clinical trials. Clinicians are invited to develop these new agents, as a broad spectrum of new drugs and advances in clinical trial methods may permit more reliable determinations of efficacy and safety and, ultimately, effectiveness in the treatment of OIC [8].

ACKNOWLEDGMENTS

The authors thank Dr. W. Hyun Song, Dr. Young Jun Eum and Ms Myung Hwa Kim for their assistance in the collection of data.

REFERENCES

[1] Ahmedzai S, Brooks D (1997) Transdermal fentanyl versus sustained-release oral morphine in cancer pain: preference, efficacy, and quality of life. The TTS-Fentanyl Comparative Trial Group. *J Pain Symptom Manage* 13: 254-261.

[2] Anderson VC, Burchiel KJ (1999) A prospective study of long-term intrathecal morphine in the management of chronic nonmalignant pain. *Neurosurgery* 44: 289-300; discussion 300-281.

[3] Angst MS, Drover DR, Lotsch J, Ramaswamy B, Naidu S, Wada DR, Stanski DR (2001) Pharmacodynamics of orally administered sustained-release hydromorphone in humans. *Anesthesiology* 94: 63-73.

[4] Benich JJ (2011) Opioid dependence. *Prim Care* 38: 59-70, vi.

[5] Binsfeld H, Szczepanski L, Waechter S, Richarz U, Sabatowski R (2010) A randomized study to demonstrate non-inferiority of once-daily OROS(®) hydromorphone with twice-daily sustained-release oxycodone for moderate to severe chronic noncancer pain. *Pain Pract* 10: 404-415.

[6] Bohnert AS, Valenstein M, Bair MJ, Ganoczy D, McCarthy JF, Ilgen MA, Blow FC (2011) Association between opioid prescribing patterns and opioid overdose-related deaths. *JAMA* 305: 1315-1321.

[7] Butts M, Jatoi A (2011) A systematic compilation of reports published on opioid-related problems. *J Opioid Manag* 7: 35-45.

[8] Camilleri M (2011) Opioid-induced constipation: challenges and therapeutic opportunities. *Am J Gastroenterol* 106: 835-842; quiz 843.

[9] Caraceni A, Pigni A, Brunelli C (2011) Is oral morphine still the first choice opioid for moderate to severe cancer pain? A systematic review within the European Palliative Care Research Collaborative guidelines project. *Palliat Med* 25: 402-409.

[10] Chaney MA (1995) Side effects of intrathecal and epidural opioids. *Can J Anaesth* 42: 891-903.

[11] Chang AK, Bijur PE, Campbell CM, Murphy MK, Gallagher EJ (2009) Safety and efficacy of rapid titration using 1mg doses of intravenous hydromorphone in emergency department patients with acute severe pain: the "1+1" protocol. *Ann Emerg Med* 54: 221-225.

[12] Chang AK, Bijur PE, Gallagher EJ (2011) Randomized Clinical Trial Comparing the Safety and Efficacy of a Hydromorphone Titration Protocol to Usual Care in the Management of Adult Emergency Department Patients With Acute Severe Pain. *Ann Emerg Med.*

[13] Chang AK, Bijur PE, Napolitano A, Lupow J, Gallagher EJ (2009) Two milligrams i.v. hydromorphone is efficacious for treating pain but is associated with oxygen desaturation. *J Opioid Manag* 5: 75-80.

[14] Choi YS, Billings JA (2002) Opioid antagonists: a review of their role in palliative care, focusing on use in opioid-related constipation. *J Pain Symptom Manage* 24: 71-90.

[15] Coluzzi F, Mattia C (2010) OROS® hydromorphone in chronic pain management: when drug delivery technology matches clinical needs. *Minerva Anestesiol* 76: 1072-1084.

[16] Coombs DW (1988) Intraspinal analgesic infusion by implanted pump. *Ann N Y Acad Sci* 531: 108-122.

[17] Cousins MJ (2007) Advances in the long-term management of chronic pain: Recent evidence with OROS (R) hydromorphone, a novel, once-daily, long-acting opioid analgesic - Introduction. *Journal of Pain and Symptom Management* 33: S1-S3.

[18] Davis MP, Varga J, Dickerson D, Walsh D, LeGrand SB, Lagman R (2003) Normal-release and controlled-release oxycodone: pharmacokinetics, pharmacodynamics, and controversy. *Support Care Cancer* 11: 84-92.

[19] Dellemijn PL, Vanneste JA (1997) Randomised double-blind active-placebo-controlled crossover trial of intravenous fentanyl in neuropathic pain. *Lancet* 349: 753-758.

[20] Di Chiro G (1966) Observations on the circulation of the cerebrospinal fluid. *Acta Radiol Diagn (Stockh)* 5: 988-1002.

[21] Diego L, Atayee R, Helmons P, Hsiao G, von Gunten CF (2011) Novel opioid antagonists for opioid-induced bowel dysfunction. *Expert Opin Investig Drugs.*

[22] Dodrill CL, Helmer DA, Kosten TR (2011) Prescription pain medication dependence. *Am J Psychiatry* 168: 466-471.

[23] Drover DR, Angst MS, Valle M, Ramaswamy B, Naidu S, Stanski DR, Verotta D (2002) Input characteristics and bioavailability after administration of immediate and a new extended-release formulation of hydromorphone in healthy volunteers. *Anesthesiology* 97: 827-836.

[24] Edgerton L, Loven B (2011) Clinical inquiries. What are the adverse effects of prolonged opioid use in patients with chronic pain? *J Fam Pract* 60: 288-289.

[25] Falk E (1917) Eukodal, ein neues Narkotikum. *Munch Med Wochenschr* 20: 381-384.

[26] Fallon MT, Laird BJ (2011) A systematic review of combination step III opioid therapy in cancer pain: An EPCRC opioid guideline project. *Palliat Med* 25: 597-603.

[27] Ferrell B, Wisdom C, Wenzl C, Brown J (1989) Effects of controlled-released morphine on quality of life for cancer pain. *Oncol Nurs Forum* 16: 521-526.

[28] Goforth HW (2010) Hydromorphone-OROS formulation. *Expert Opin Pharmacother* 11: 1207-1214.

[29] Goldstein A, Lowney LI, Pal BK (1971) Stereospecific and nonspecific interactions of the morphine congener levorphanol in subcellular fractions of mouse brain. *Proc Natl Acad Sci U S A* 68: 1742-1747.

[30] Gourlay GK, Kowalski SR, Plummer JL, Cherry DA, Gaukroger P, Cousins MJ (1989) The transdermal administration of fentanyl in the treatment of postoperative pain: pharmacokinetics and pharmacodynamic effects. *Pain* 37: 193-202.

[31] Gupta SK, Southam M, Gale R, Hwang SS (1992) System functionality and physicochemical model of fentanyl transdermal system. *J Pain Symptom Manage* 7: S17-26.

[32] Hale M, Khan A, Kutch M, Li S (2010) Once-daily OROS hydromorphone ER compared with placebo in opioid-tolerant patients with chronic low back pain. *Curr Med Res Opin* 26: 1505-1518.

[33] Hale M, Upmalis D, Okamoto A, Lange C, Rauschkolb C (2009) Tolerability of tapentadol immediate release in patients with lower back pain or osteoarthritis of the hip or knee over 90 days: a randomized, double-blind study. *Curr Med Res Opin* 25: 1095-1104.

[34] Han J, Cui C, Wu L (2011) Acupuncture-related techniques for the treatment of opiate addiction: a case of translational medicine. *Front Med* 5: 141-150.

[35] Handal KA, Schauben JL, Salamone FR (1983) Naloxone. *Ann Emerg Med* 12: 438-445.

[36] Hanks GW, Conno F, Cherny N, Hanna M, Kalso E, McQuay HJ, Mercadante S, Meynadier J, Poulain P, Ripamonti C, Radbruch L, Casas JR, Sawe J, Twycross RG, Ventafridda V (2001) Morphine and alternative opioids in cancer pain: the EAPC recommendations. *Br J Cancer* 84: 587-593.

[37] Hartrick C, Van Hove I, Stegmann JU, Oh C, Upmalis D (2009) Efficacy and tolerability of tapentadol immediate release and oxycodone HCl immediate release in patients awaiting primary joint replacement surgery for end-stage joint disease: a 10-day, phase III, randomized, double-blind, active- and placebo-controlled study. *Clin Ther* 31: 260-271.

[38] Hartrick CT (2010) Tapentadol immediate-release for acute pain. *Expert Rev Neurother* 10: 861-869.

[39] Hassenbusch SJ, Pillay PK, Magdinec M, Currie K, Bay JW, Covington EC, Tomaszewski MZ (1990) Constant infusion of morphine for intractable cancer pain using an implanted pump. *J Neurosurg* 73: 405-409.

[40] Hassenbusch SJ, Stanton-Hicks M, Covington EC, Walsh JG, Guthrey DS (1995) Long-term intraspinal infusions of opioids in the treatment of neuropathic pain. *J Pain Symptom Manage* 10: 527-543.

[41] Herbst LH, Strause LG (1992) Transdermal fentanyl use in hospice home-care patients with chronic cancer pain. *J Pain Symptom Manage* 7: S54-57.

[42] Holley FO, van Steennis C (1988) Postoperative analgesia with fentanyl: pharmacokinetics and pharmacodynamics of constant-rate i.v. and transdermal delivery. *Br J Anaesth* 60: 608-613.

[43] Hovaguimian A, Gibbons CH (2011) Clinical Approach to the Treatment of Painful Diabetic Neuropathy. *Ther Adv Endocrinol Metab* 2: 27-38.

[44] Kaplan R, Parris WC, Citron ML, Zhukovsky D, Reder RF, Buckley BJ, Kaiko RF (1998) Comparison of controlled-release and immediate-release oxycodone tablets in patients with cancer pain. *J Clin Oncol* 16: 3230-3237.

[45] Karst M, Fink M, Wagner T, Conrad I (2001) Transdermal fentanyl: little absorption in two patients with systemic sclerosis? *Pain Med* 2: 225-227.

[46] King SJ, Reid C, Forbes K, Hanks G (2011) A systematic review of oxycodone in the management of cancer pain. *Palliat Med* 25: 454-470.

[47] Klepstad P, Kaasa S, Borchgrevink PC (2011) Starting Step III opioids for moderate to severe pain in cancer patients: Dose titration: A systematic review. *Palliat Med* 25: 424-430.

[48] Koulousakis A, Kuchta J, Bayarassou A, Sturm V (2007) Intrathecal opioids for intractable pain syndromes. *Acta Neurochir Suppl* 97: 43-48.

[49] Krames ES (1993) Intrathecal infusional therapies for intractable pain: patient management guidelines. *J Pain Symptom Manage* 8: 36-46.

[50] Kurz A, Sessler DI (2003) Opioid-induced bowel dysfunction: pathophysiology and potential new therapies. *Drugs* 63: 649-671.

[51] Lalovic B, Kharasch E, Hoffer C, Risler L, Liu-Chen LY, Shen DD (2006) Pharmacokinetics and pharmacodynamics of oral oxycodone in healthy human subjects: role of circulating active metabolites. *Clin Pharmacol Ther* 79: 461-479.

[52] LaMotte CC, Snowman A, Pert CB, Synder SH (1978) Opiate receptor binding in rhesus monkey brain: association with limbic structures. *Brain Res* 155: 374-379.

[53] Larsen RH, Nielsen F, Sørensen JA, Nielsen JB (2003) Dermal penetration of fentanyl: inter- and intraindividual variations. *Pharmacol Toxicol* 93: 244-248.

[54] Lehmann KA, Zech D (1992) Transdermal fentanyl: clinical pharmacology. *J Pain Symptom Manage* 7: S8-16.

[55] Linares OA, Linares AL (2011) Computational opioid prescribing: a novel application of clinical pharmacokinetics. *J Pain Palliat Care Pharmacother* 25: 125-135.

[56] Ling W, Mooney L, Hillhouse M (2011) Prescription opioid abuse, pain and addiction: clinical issues and implications. *Drug Alcohol Rev* 30: 300-305.

[57] Lipman AG, Karver S, Austin Cooney G, Stambler N, Israel RJ (2011) Methylnaltrexone for opioid-induced constipation in patients with advanced illness: a 3-month open-label treatment extension study. *J Pain Palliat Care Pharmacother* 25: 136-145.

[58] Lowenstein O, Leyendecker P, Lux EA, Blagden M, Simpson KH, Hopp M, Bosse B, Reimer K (2010) Efficacy and safety of combined prolonged-release oxycodone and naloxone in the management of moderate/severe chronic non-malignant pain: results of a prospectively designed pooled analysis of two randomised, double-blind clinical trials. *BMC Clin Pharmacol* 10: 12.

[59] Machelska H (2011) *Control of Neuropathic Pain by Immune Cells and Opioids*. CNS Neurol Disord Drug Targets.

[60] Manchikanti L, Ailinani H, Koyyalagunta D, Datta S, Singh V, Eriator I, Sehgal N, Shah R, Benyamin R, Vallejo R, Fellows B, Christo PJ (2011) A systematic review of randomized trials of long-term opioid management for chronic non-cancer pain. *Pain Physician* 14: 91-121.

[61] Manchikanti L, Vallejo R, Manchikanti KN, Benyamin RM, Datta S, Christo PJ (2011) Effectiveness of long-term opioid therapy for chronic non-cancer pain. *Pain Physician* 14: E133-156.

[62] Meissner W, Leyendecker P, Mueller-Lissner S, Nadstawek J, Hopp M, Ruckes C, Wirz S, Fleischer W, Reimer K (2009) A randomised controlled trial with prolonged-release oral oxycodone and naloxone to prevent and reverse opioid-induced constipation. *Eur J Pain* 13: 56-64.

[63] Meyer MR, Maurer HH (2011) Absorption, distribution, metabolism and excretion pharmacogenomics of drugs of abuse. *Pharmacogenomics* 12: 215-233.

[64] Minozzi S, Amato L, Vecchi S, Davoli M, Kirchmayer U, Verster A (2011) *Oral naltrexone maintenance treatment for opioid dependence*. Cochrane Database Syst Rev: CD001333.

[65] Moore KT, St-Fleur D, Marricco NC, Ariyawansa J, Page V, Natarajan J, Morelli G, Richarz U (2010) Steady-state pharmacokinetics of extended-release hydromorphone (OROS hydromorphone): a randomized study in healthy volunteers. *J Opioid Manag* 6: 351-358.

[66] Murray A, Hagen NA (2005) Hydromorphone. *J Pain Symptom Manage* 29: S57-66.

[67] Nelson L, Schwaner R (2009) Transdermal fentanyl: pharmacology and toxicology. *J Med Toxicol* 5: 230-241.

[68] Newshan G, Lefkowitz M (2001) Transdermal fentanyl for chronic pain in AIDS: a pilot study. *J Pain Symptom Manage* 21: 69-77.

[69] Okie S (2010) A flood of opioids, a rising tide of deaths. *N Engl J Med* 363: 1981-1985.

[70] Onofrio BM, Yaksh TL (1990) Long-term pain relief produced by intrathecal morphine infusion in 53 patients. *J Neurosurg* 72: 200-209.

[71] Onofrio BM, Yaksh TL, Arnold PG (1981) Continuous low-dose intrathecal morphine administration in the treatment of chronic pain of malignant origin. *Mayo Clin Proc* 56: 516-520.

[72] Pan H, Zhang Z, Zhang Y, Xu N, Lu L, Dou C, Guo Y, Wu S, Yue J, Wu D, Dai Y (2007) Efficacy and tolerability of oxycodone hydrochloride controlled-release tablets in moderate to severe cancer pain. *Clin Drug Investig* 27: 259-267.

[73] Panchal SJ, Muller-Schwefe P, Wurzelmann JI (2007) Opioid-induced bowel dysfunction: prevalence, pathophysiology and burden. *Int J Clin Pract* 61: 1181-1187.

[74] Pappagallo M (2001) Incidence, prevalence, and management of opioid bowel dysfunction. *Am J Surg* 182: 11S-18S.

[75] Park JH, Kim JH, Yun SC, Roh SW, Rhim SC, Kim CJ, Jeon SR (2011) Evaluation of efficacy and safety of fentanyl transdermal patch (Durogesic D-TRANS) in chronic pain. *Acta Neurochir (Wien)* 153: 181-190.

[76] Patt RB, Hogan LA (1992) Transdermal fentanyl for chronic cancer pain: detailed case reports and the influence of confounding factors. *J Pain Symptom Manage* 7: S51-53.

[77] Payne R (1992) Transdermal fentanyl: suggested recommendations for clinical use. *J Pain Symptom Manage* 7: S40-44.

[78] Payne R, Mathias SD, Pasta DJ, Wanke LA, Williams R, Mahmoud R (1998) Quality of life and cancer pain: satisfaction and side effects with transdermal fentanyl versus oral morphine. *J Clin Oncol* 16: 1588-1593.

[79] Penn RD, Paice JA (1987) Chronic intrathecal morphine for intractable pain. *J Neurosurg* 67: 182-186.

[80] Pigni A, Brunelli C, Caraceni A (2011) The role of hydromorphone in cancer pain treatment: a systematic review. *Palliat Med* 25: 471-477.

[81] Portenoy RK, Southam MA, Gupta SK, Lapin J, Layman M, Inturrisi CE, Foley KM (1993) Transdermal fentanyl for cancer pain. Repeated dose pharmacokinetics. *Anesthesiology* 78: 36-43.

[82] Poyhia R, Vainio A, Kalso E (1993) A review of oxycodone's clinical pharmacokinetics and pharmacodynamics. *J Pain Symptom Manage* 8: 63-67.

[83] Reder RF, Oshlack B, Miotto JB, Benziger DD, Kaiko RF (1996) Steady-state bioavailability of controlled-release oxycodone in normal subjects. *Clin Ther* 18: 95-105.

[84] Resine T PG (1995) Opioid analgesics and antagonists. In: *Goodman & Gilman's The Pharmacological Basis of Therapeutics.* 9th ed. Hardman JG, Limbird LE,Molinoff PB, et al, eds, New York, NY: McGraw-Hill, pp 521-555.

[85] Riley J, Eisenberg E, Muller-Schwefe G, Drewes AM, Arendt-Nielsen L (2008) Oxycodone: a review of its use in the management of pain. *Curr Med Res Opin* 24: 175-192.

[86] Roland CL, Setnik B, Cleveland JM, Brown DA (2011) Clinical outcomes during opioid titration following initiation with or conversion to Remoxy®, an extended-release formulation of oxycodone. *Postgrad Med* 123: 148-159.

[87] Ross JR, Quigley C (2003) Transdermal fentanyl: informed prescribing is essential. *Eur J Pain* 7: 481-483.

[88] Salzman RT, Roberts MS, Wild J, Fabian C, Reder RF, Goldenheim PD (1999) Can a controlled-release oral dose form of oxycodone be used as readily as an immediate-release form for the purpose of titrating to stable pain control? *J Pain Symptom Manage* 18: 271-279.

[89] Sarhill N, Walsh D, Nelson KA (2001) Hydromorphone: pharmacology and clinical applications in cancer patients. *Support Care Cancer* 9: 84-96.

[90] Savage SR (1996) Long-term opioid therapy: assessment of consequences and risks. *J Pain Symptom Manage* 11: 274-286.

[91] Sawe J (1986) High-dose morphine and methadone in cancer patients. Clinical pharmacokinetic considerations of oral treatment. *Clin Pharmacokinet* 11: 87-106.

[92] Schneider JP, Matthews M, Jamison RN (2010) Abuse-deterrent and tamper-resistant opioid formulations: what is their role in addressing prescription opioid abuse? *CNS Drugs* 24: 805-810.

[93] Schultheiss R, Schramm J, Neidhardt J (1992) Dose changes in long- and medium-term intrathecal morphine therapy of cancer pain. *Neurosurgery* 31: 664-669; discussion 669-670.

[94] Shram MJ, Sathyan G, Khanna S, Tudor IC, Nath R, Thipphawong J, Sellers EM (2010) Evaluation of the abuse potential of extended release hydromorphone versus immediate release hydromorphone. *J Clin Psychopharmacol* 30: 25-33.

[95] Simmonds MA, Richenbacher J (1992) Transdermal fentanyl: long-term analgesic studies. *J Pain Symptom Manage* 7: S36-39.

[96] Siniscalchi A, Gallelli L, Avenoso T, Squillace A, De Sarro G (2011) Effects of carbamazepine/oxycodone coadministration in the treatment of trigeminal neuralgia. *Ann Pharmacother* 45: e33.

[97] Slover R (1992) Transdermal fentanyl: clinical trial at the University of Colorado Health Sciences Center. *J Pain Symptom Manage* 7: S45-47.

[98] Smith K, Hopp M, Mundin G, Leyendecker P, Bailey P, Grothe B, Uhl R, Reimer K (2008) Single- and multiple-dose pharmacokinetic evaluation of oxycodone and naloxone in an opioid agonist/antagonist prolonged-release combination in healthy adult volunteers. *Clin Ther* 30: 2051-2068.

[99] Solassol I, Bressolle F, Caumette L, Garcia F, Poujol S, Culine S, Pinguet F (2005) Inter- and intraindividual variabilities in pharmacokinetics of fentanyl after repeated 72-hour transdermal applications in cancer pain patients. *Ther Drug Monit* 27: 491-498.

[100] Stambaugh JE, Reder RF, Stambaugh MD, Stambaugh H, Davis M (2001) Double-blind, randomized comparison of the analgesic and pharmacokinetic profiles of controlled- and immediate-release oral oxycodone in cancer pain patients. *J Clin Pharmacol* 41: 500-506.

[101] Stanley TH (1992) The history and development of the fentanyl series. *J Pain Symptom Manage* 7: S3-7.

[102] Stepanovi? A, Pirc J, Lahajnar ?avlovi? S (2011) *Clinical efficacy of OROS(®) hydromorphone in patients suffering from severe chronic pain: A Study undertaken in routine clinical practice.* Wien Klin Wochenschr.

[103] Tessaro L, Bandieri E, Costa G, Fornasier G, Iorno V, Pizza C, Pastacaldi G, Micheletto G (2010) Use of oxycodone controlled-release immediately after NSAIDs: a new approach to obtain good pain control. *Eur Rev Med Pharmacol Sci* 14: 113-121.

[104] TJB (1999) *Pain Management.* McGraw-Hill Medical Publishing Division, New York, NY.

[105] Trescot AM, Helm S, Hansen H, Benyamin R, Glaser SE, Adlaka R, Patel S, Manchikanti L (2008) Opioids in the management of chronic non-cancer pain: an update of American Society of the Interventional Pain Physicians' (ASIPP) *Guidelines. Pain Physician* 11: S5-S62.

[106] Turgeon J, Groning R, Sathyan G, Thipphawong J, Richarz U (2010) The pharmacokinetics of a long-acting OROS hydromorphone formulation. *Expert Opin Drug Deliv* 7: 137-144.

[107] Tzschentke TM, Christoph T, Kogel B, Schiene K, Hennies HH, Englberger W, Haurand M, Jahnel U, Cremers TI, Friderichs E, De Vry J (2007) (-)-(1R,2R)-3-(3-dimethylamino-1-ethyl-2-methyl-propyl)-phenol hydrochloride (tapentadol HCl): a

novel mu-opioid receptor agonist/norepinephrine reuptake inhibitor with broad-spectrum analgesic properties. *J Pharmacol Exp Ther* 323: 265-276.

[108] Tzschentke TM, De Vry J, Terlinden R, Hennies HH, Lange C, Strassburger W, Haurand M, Kolb J, Schneider J, Buschmann H, Finkam M, Jahnel U (2006) Tapentadol hydrochloride. Analgesic, Mu-opioid receptor agonist, noradrenaline reuptake inhibitor. *Drugs of the Future* 31: 1053-1061.

[109] Tzschentke TM, Jahnel U, Kogel B, Christoph T, Englberger W, De Vry J, Schiene K, Okamoto A, Upmalis D, Weber H, Lange C, Stegmann JU, Kleinert R (2009) Tapentadol hydrochloride: a next-generation, centrally acting analgesic with two mechanisms of action in a single molecule. *Drugs Today (Barc)* 45: 483-496.

[110] Varvel JR, Shafer SL, Hwang SS, Coen PA, Stanski DR (1989) Absorption characteristics of transdermally administered fentanyl. *Anesthesiology* 70: 928-934.

[111] Vondrackova D, Leyendecker P, Meissner W, Hopp M, Szombati I, Hermanns K, Ruckes C, Weber S, Grothe B, Fleischer W, Reimer K (2008) Analgesic efficacy and safety of oxycodone in combination with naloxone as prolonged release tablets in patients with moderate to severe chronic pain. *J Pain* 9: 1144-1154.

[112] Wu CL, Raja SN (2011) Treatment of acute postoperative pain. *The Lancet* 377: 2215-2225.

[113] Yaksh TL (1984) Multiple opioid receptor systems in brain and spinal cord: Part 2. *Eur J Anaesthesiol* 1: 201-243.

[114] Yaksh TL (1984) Multiple opioid receptor systems in brain and spinal cord: Part I. *Eur J Anaesthesiol* 1: 171-199.

[115] Yaksh TL, Rudy TA (1976) Analgesia mediated by a direct spinal action of narcotics. *Science* 192: 1357-1358.

[116] Zeppetella G (2011) Opioids for the management of breakthrough cancer pain in adults: A systematic review undertaken as part of an EPCRC opioid guidelines project. *Palliat Med* 25: 516-524.

In: Opioids: Pharmacology, Clinical Uses and Adverse Effects ISBN 978-1-61942-101-1
Editors: Djavakhi Tvildiani and Kakha Gegechkori

Chapter 7

ASSOCIATION BETWEEN ANALGESIC REQUIREMENTS AFTER MAJOR ABDOMINAL SURGERY AND POLYMORPHISMS OF THE OPIOIDMETABOLISM-RELATED GENE ABCB1

Daisuke Kobayashi[1,2,*], Daisuke Nishizawa[1,*], Shinya Kasai[1], Junko Hasegawa[1], Makoto Nagashima[3], Ryoji Katoh[3], Yasuo Satoh[4], Megumi Tagami[4], Masakazu Hayashida[5], Kenichi Fukuda[2] and Kazutaka Ikeda[1#]

Division of Psychobiology, Tokyo Institute of Psychiatry, Tokyo, Japan[1]
Department of Clinical Oral Health Science, Tokyo Dental College, Suidoubashi Hospital, Tokyo, Japan[2]
Department of Surgery, Toho University Sakura Medical Center, Sakura, Japan[3]
Department of Anesthesiology, Toho University Sakura Medical Center, Sakura, Japan[4]
Department of Anesthesiology, Saitama Medical University International Medical Center, Hidaka, Japan[5]

ABSTRACT

Analyses of opioid.-related molecules using genetically modified animals have clarified the mechanisms of the analgesic action of morphine, its related side-effects, and individual variabilities in sensitivity. In the present study, we examined the relationship between the dosage of analgesics, including opioids, required after major abdominal surgery and polymorphisms of an opioid metabolism-related gene, ATP-binding cassette, sub-family B (MDR/TAP), member 1 (*ABCB1*). We studied 129 patients (74 males, 55 females; aged 28-80 years old) who were administered analgesics, including opioids, for

* These authors contributed equally to this study.
# Corresponding author: Kazutaka Ikeda, Ph.D., Director, Molecular Psychiatry Research Tokyo Institute of Psychiatry, 2-1-8 Kamikitazawa, Setagaya-ku, Tokyo 156-8585, Japan, Phone: +81-3-3304-5701; Fax: +81-3-3329-8035; E-mail: ikedak@prit.go.jp.

pain relief following major abdominal surgery and who provided informed consent. The analyses were performed using multivariate analysis, with $p < 0.05$ considered statistically significant. We found a significant association between analgesic requirements and *ABCB1* polymorphisms. Studies on gene polymorphisms associated with analgesic requirements are important for developing appropriate personalized treatments with less side-effects.

1. Introduction

Opioids are commonly used as effective analgesics for the treatment of acute and chronic pain. However, sensitivity to opioid analgesics is well known to vary widely among individual subjects [1]. Because of this variability, a dose of an opioid analgesic that can produce satisfactory pain relief without adverse effects in some patients might cause under-dosing or overdosing in other patients. Among opioid-related genes, the μ-opioid receptor gene is the major candidate gene for investigation [2] because μ-opioid receptor knockout mice display abolished morphine-induced analgesia in several tests of nociceptive responsiveness [3]. Recently, several studies in humans have revealed a relationship between genetic variations in the μ-opioid receptor gene and sensitivity to opioid analgesics [4-8].

An opioid metabolism-related gene, ATP-binding cassette, sub-family B (MDR/TAP), member 1 (*ABCB1*), encodes a blood-brain barrier transporter P-glycoprotein that plays an important role in controlling substance passage between the blood and brain. Thus, the ABCB1 protein reportedly plays a role in morphine metabolism [9]. Genetic variations in the human *ABCB1* gene have been the most extensively studied. More than 50 single nucleotide polymorphisms (SNPs) and insertion/deletion polymorphisms in the *ABCB1* gene have been reported. However, information is still limited with respect to the actual effects of these genetic polymorphisms on the function of the ABCB1 protein. In the present study, we examined the possible association of three *ABCB1* polymorphisms with sensitivity to opioid that have been reportedly associated with methadone requirements, an opioid used in heroin dependence treatment.

2. Methods

2.1. Subjects

One hundred twenty-nine patients participated in the association study. Subjects had undergone major open abdominal surgery, mostly gastrectomy for gastric cancer and colectomy for colorectal cancer, under combined general and epidural anesthesia at Research Hospital, Institute of Medical Science, The University of Tokyo, or at Toho University Sakura Medical Center. Peripheral blood or oral mucosa samples were collected from these subjects for gene analysis.

The study protocol was approved by the Institutional Review Boards at the Institute of Medical Science, The University of Tokyo (Tokyo, Japan), Toho University Sakura Medical Center (Sakura, Japan), and the Tokyo Institute of Psychiatry (Tokyo, Japan). All subjects provided informed, written consent for the genetics studies.

2.2. Clinical Data

Postoperative pain was managed primarily with continuous epidural analgesia with fentanyl or morphine. Fentanyl or morphine was diluted with 0.25% bupivacaine in a total volume of 100 ml and infused through the catheter placed in the lower thoracic or upper lumbar epidural space at a constant rate of 2 ml/h. Whenever the patient complained of significant postoperative pain despite continuous epidural analgesic, appropriate doses of opioids, including buprenorphine, pentazocine, and pethidine, and/or nonsteroidal anti-inflammatory drugs (NSAIDs), including diclofenac, flurbiprofen, and indomethacin, were systemically administered as rescue analgesics at the discretion of surgeons. Also, epidural morphine was administered in some patients. The clinical data sampled included age, gender, body height, body weight, postoperative diagnosis, type of operation, duration of operation, and frequency and doses of rescue analgesics (opioids and/or NSAIDs) administered during the first 24 h postoperative period, for which analgesic therapy would be required in most patients.

To allow intersubject comparisons of rescue analgesic doses required during the first 24 h postoperative period, doses of opioids and NSAIDs administered as rescue analgesics during this period were converted to the equivalent dose of systemic pentazocine. The dose of epidural morphine required for pain relief after abdominal surgery is approximately one-fifth that of systemic morphine [10]. Systemic pentazocine is one-third as potent as systemic morphine, and systemic buprenorphine is approximately 30-times as potent as systemic morphine [11]. Systemic flurbiprofen, diclofenac, and indomethacin are equivalent [12, 13]. The analgesic effect of systemic diclofenac, 1 mg/kg, is comparable to that of systemic fentanyl, 1 μg/kg [14, 15]. Systemic fentanyl is 100-times more potent than systemic morphine [16]. Therefore, systemic buprenorphine, 400 μg was converted to the equivalent systemic pentazocine dose of 30 mg in this study. As systemic pethidine is considered to be less potent than systemic morphine, 35 mg systemic pethidine was converted to the equivalent systemic morphine dose of 10 mg and thus systemic pentazocine dose of 30 mg. Systemic flurbiprofen, 50 mg, and systemic diclofenac, 50 mg, and systemic indomethacin, 50 mg, were converted to the equivalent systemic pentazocine dose of 15 mg. The frequency of rescue analgesic administration was determined as the frequency of the use of rescue analgesics during the first 24 h postoperative period. The total dose of rescue analgesics administered was determined as the sum of systemic pentazocine-equivalent doses of all opioids and NSAIDs given to patients as rescue analgesics during the same period.

2.3. Genotyping

Total genomic DNA was extracted from peripheral blood samples by standard procedures. For genotyping rs1128503, the polymerase chain reaction-restriction fragment length polymorphism (PCR-RFLP) method was adopted. To perform PCR-RFLP, the restriction enzyme EcoO109I (Takara K.K. Japan, Shiga, Japan) and two primers of H44 and H45 were used (Table 1).

First, PCR was performed in a final volume of 10 μl containing 5× GoTaq™ reaction buffer (Promega K.K. Japan, Tokyo, Japan), 0.8 mM dioxyribonucleoside triphosphate, 0.5

μM of each primer, 0.05 U GoTaq™ DNA polymerase (Promega), and 5-50 ng extracted genomic DNA as the template. The PCR program was the following: 95°C for 1 min, followed by 35 cycles of 95°C for 30 s, 60°C for 30 s, and 72°C for 1 min, with a final extension at 72°C for 5 min. The amplified DNA fragments were digested by the restriction enzyme at 37°C in a total of 10 μl reaction solution containing 10× L Buffer, 0.75 U EcoO109I (Takara K.K. Japan, Shiga, Japan), and 5 μl PCR product as the substrate.

Table 1. Primers used in the analyses of ABCB1 polymorphisms

rsID	Sequence	Forward/Reverse	Primer No.
1128503	ATCCAGCTCTCCACAAAATATCATAAAG	Forward	H44
	CTGATCACCGCAGGGTCTAGCTCGCATGG GTCCTC	Reverse	H45
1045642	ACACAAACTTTTCCTTAATCTCACAG	Forward	H51
	TTTGGTTGCTAATTTCTCTTCACTTC	Reverse	H52
2032582	ACTCTTAGCAATTGTACCCATCAT	Forward	H46
	AAACACATTCTTAGAGCATAGT	Reverse	H50

The digestion products were analyzed by electrophoresis using 1-2% agarose gel and ethidium bromide staining for visualization under ultraviolet illumination. The appearance of both the 366 bp and 134 bp DNA fragments of the loaded sample corresponded to the C/C genotype. The appearance of the 490 bp, 366 bp, and 134 bp fragments corresponded to the T/C genotype, and the appearance of the 490 bp fragment corresponded to the T/T genotype.

For genotyping rs1045642, the PCR-RFLP method was also adopted. To perform PCR-RFLP, the restriction enzyme Mbo I and two primers of H51 and H52 were used (Table 1). First, PCR was performed in a final volume of 10 μl containing 2× GoTaq™ Master Mix (Promega), 0.5 μM of each primer, and 5-50 ng extracted genomic DNA as the template. The PCR program was the following: 95°C for 1 min, followed by 35 cycles of 95°C for 30 s, 55°C for 30 s, and 72°C for 1 min, with a final extension at 72°C for 5 min. The amplified DNA fragments were digested by the restriction enzyme at 37°C in a total of 10 μl reaction solution containing 10× K Buffer (Takara), 1 U MboI (Takara), and 5 μl PCR product as the substrate. The digestion products were analyzed by electrophoresis using 1-2% agarose gel and ethidium bromide staining for visualization under ultraviolet illumination. The appearance of the 172 bp, 169 bp, and 98 bp DNA fragments of the loaded sample corresponded to the C/C genotype. The appearance of the 341 bp, 172 bp, 169 bp, and 98 bp fragments corresponded to the T/C genotype, and the appearance of the 341 bp and 98 bp fragments corresponded to the T/T genotype.

For genotyping rs2032582, direct sequencing was adopted. To perform direct sequencing, two primers of H46 and H50 were used (Table 1). First, PCR was performed in a final volume of 10 μl containing 2× GoTaq™ Master Mix (Promega), 0.5 μM of each primer, and 5-50 ng extracted genomic DNA as the template. The PCR program was the following: 95°C for 1 min, followed by 35 cycles of 95°C for 30 s, 50°C for 30 s, and 72°C for 1 min, with a final extension at 72°C for 5 min. Following the cycle sequencing reaction with the BigDye® Terminator version 3.1 Cycle Sequencing Kit (Applied Biosystems Japan, Tokyo, Japan) according to the manufacturer's instructions and purification of the PCR products, DNA sequences of the fragments were determined using the automated sequencer ABI PRISM® 3100 Genetic Analyzer (Applied Biosystems Japan) with both forward and reverse primers.

2.4. Statistical Analysis

The χ^2 test was performed for all genotype frequency data using FreeJSTAT 8.2 for Windows (free software by M. Sato, Japan; current version is available at http://www. vector.co /win95/b.jp/soft usiness/se030917.html; accessed October 13, 2008) to investigate the deviation of the distributions from those in the theoretical Hardy-Weinberg equilibrium. Analysis of variance (ANOVA) was performed to examine the contribution of the SNPs to the frequency of 24 h analgesic requirements and postoperative 24 h analgesic requirements. ANOVA was performed using SPSS (12.0J for Windows, SPSS Japan, Tokyo, Japan). Power analyses were performed using G*Power version 3.0.5 [17]. Values of $p < 0.05$ were considered statistically significant.

3. Results

The clinical data of the 129 subjects who were included in the association study are provided in Table 2. Rescue analgesics were required in 72 patients. Doses of rescue analgesics administered to patients are shown in Table 2. The allele frequencies in these SNPs were similar to those in a previous report [18] (Table 3). The genotype distributions for the three SNPs selected were not significantly different from the theoretical values of Hardy-Weinberg equilibrium (data not shown).

Two-way ANOVA was performed to examine the effects of SNPs and gender on the frequency of rescue analgesic administration and the total dose of rescue analgesics administered. Statistical power analyses for the ANOVA revealed that the expected power (1 minus type II error probability) was 71% for the Cohen's conventional "medium" effect size 0.25 [19] when the sample size was 129 and type I error probability was set at 0.05. Significant associations were not observed between rs1045642 and rs2032582 and the frequency of rescue analgesic administration and total dose of rescue analgesics administered (data not shown). Significant associations were not observed between the three SNPs and total dose of rescue analgesics administered after Bonferroni correction. However, a significant main effect of the *ABCB1* rs1128503 SNP on the frequency of rescue analgesic administration was found when the C/C genotype was compared with the combined C/T and T/T genotypes ($F_{1, 125} = 6.283$, $p = 0.013$; Figure 1). This difference was significant even after Bonferroni correction for the three SNPs ($p = 0.039$), indicating that the carriers of the C/C genotype required less frequent rescue analgesics compared with carriers of the C/T or T/T genotype.

Table 2. Clinical data of subjects included in the study

	N	Minimum	Maximum	Mean	SD
Gender					
male	74				
female	55				
Age	129	28	80	63.57	9.92
Height (cm)	129	133	175	158.21	8.34
Weight (kg)	129	35	80	56.24	10.42
Frequency of analgesic administration	129	0	8	0.95	1.18
Total dose of rescue analgesics (mg)	129	0	112.5	14.07	18.56
Epidural morphine (mg)	2	0.5	2	1.2526.25	1.06
Systemic pentazocine (mg)	24	15	75		17.83
Systemic buprenophine (mg)	15	0.2	0.8	0.47	0.16
Systemic petidine (mg)	2	17.5	35	26.25	12.37
Systemic diclofenac (mg)	24	25	100	39.58	19.39
Systemic flurbiprofen (mg)	12	50	150	62.50	31.08
Systemic indomethacin (mg)	4	25	50	43.75	12.5

Table 3. Genotype and allele frequency of ABCB1 polymorphisms

rs1128503(1236T/C)			rs2032582(2677G/T/A)			rs1045642(3435C/T)		
t	N	frequency	Genotype	N	frequency	Genotype	N	frequency
C/C	25	0.194	A/A	7	0.054	C/C	52	0.403
C/T	52	0.403	A/G	23	0.178	C/T	51	0.395
T/T	52	0.403	A/T	18	0.136	T/T	26	0.202
			G/G	23	0.178			
			G/T	30	0.233			
			T/T	27	0.209			
total	12 9	1.000	total	129	1.000	total	129	1.000
Allele frequency			Allele frequency			Allele frequency		
C	10 2	0.395	A	55	0.213	C	155	0.601
T	15 6	0.605	G	99	0.384	T	103	0.399
			T	102	0.395			
total	25 8	1.000	total	258	1.000	total	258	1.000

4. Discussion

Genetic variations of the human *ABCB1* gene have been the most extensively studied. More than 50 SNPs and insertion/deletion polymorphisms in the *ABCB1* gene have been reported. However, information is still limited with respect to the actual effect of these genetic polymorphisms on the function of the ABCB1 protein.

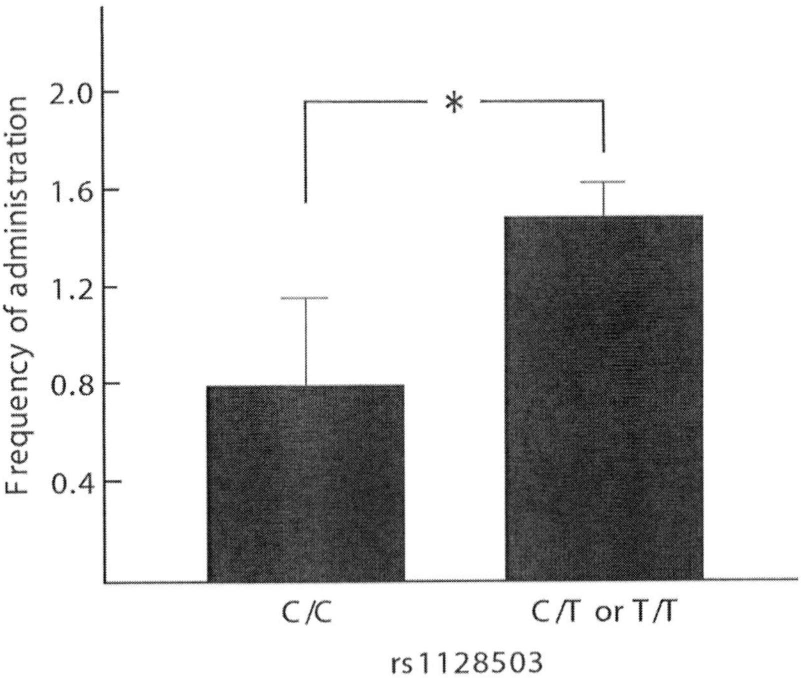

Figure 1. Association between frequency of rescue analgesic administration and *ABCB1* rs1128503. The data are presented as mean ± SEM. Asterisk indicates significant difference (*$p < 0.05$).

In the present study, we analyzed three *ABCB1* gene polymorphisms in a Japanese population who underwent major open abdominal surgery under combined general and epidural anesthesia. Previous studies have reported associations between the rs1045642, rs2032582, and rs1128503 SNPs and methadone doses required for effective treatment of heroin dependence [20].

Methadone is a μ-opioid receptor agonist used for treating opiate dependence and is also a substrate of the transporter P-glycoprotein that is encoded by the *ABCB1* gene, similar to other opioids. Therefore, we chose these three *ABCB1* SNPs for the present association study.

We found associations between the *ABCB1* gene polymorphism (rs1128503) and frequency of rescue analgesic administration. A significant main effect of the *ABCB1* rs1128503 SNP on the frequency of rescue analgesic administration was observed when the C/C genotype was compared with the combined C/T and T/T genotypes (Figure 1). Blood levels of opioids are reported to depend on the activity of the ABCB1 protein, and the activity of the ABCB1 protein in patients requiring more rescue analgesics may be higher than in other patients. This hypothesis suggests that the activity of the ABCB1 protein in patients with the C/C genotype may be lower than in patients with the C/T and T/T genotypes. rs1128503 is a synonymous variant that does not result in a change in amino acid sequence. It is located in exon 12 and within one of the intracellular loops of the protein, adjacent to an ATP-binding/utilization domain. rs1128503 may affect translation regulation, RNA stability, or other molecular mechanisms.

For our ANOVA, the desirable sample size was calculated as 158 for the effect size 0.25 to achieve 80% power. This suggests that the sample size of 129 in the present study might be insufficient to detect reliably moderate differences between the SNP genotypes. Further investigations with larger samples may reveal further associations between the *ABCB1* polymorphism and sensitivity to opioids.

In the present study, the data from patients who received NSAIDs not as main analgesics, but rather as rescue analgesics, were also analyzed. The amount of NSAIDs administered as rescue analgesics during the 24 h postoperative period were converted to the equivalent dose of systemic pentazocine. This study, therefore, investigated the relationship between *ABCB1* polymorphisms and sensitivity to opioids, not NSAIDs.

Conclusion

The present study analyzed *ABCB1* polymorphisms (rs1045642, rs2032582, rs1128503) in a Japanese population who underwent major open abdominal surgery under combined general and epidural anesthesia. We found an association between the *ABCB1* gene polymorphism rs1128503 and frequency of rescue analgesic administration. This study suggests that specific ABCB1 variants may have clinical relevance by influencing the opioid doses required. The present findings will contribute to future personalized pain treatment.

Acknowledgments

We acknowledge Mr. Michael Arends for his assistance with editing the manuscript. We are grateful to the volunteers for their participation in this study and the anesthesiologists and surgeons at Research Hospital, Institute of Medical Science, The University of Tokyo, and Toho University Sakura Medical Center for collecting clinical data. This work was supported by grants from the Ministry of Health, Labour and Welfare of Japan (H17-Pharmaco-001, H19-Iyaku-023), the Ministry of Education, Culture, Sports, Science and Technology of Japan (20602020, 19659405, 20390162), The Naito Foundation, and The Mitsubishi Foundation. The authors declare no conflict of interest.

Reviewed by

Drs. Ichiro Sora (Tohoku University Graduate School of Medicine) and Soichiro Ide (Hokkaido University Graduate School of Pharmaceutical Sciences).

References

[1] Ikeda K, Ide S, Han W, Hayashida M, Uhl GR, Sora I. *How individual sensitivity to opiates can be predicted by gene analyses.* Trends Pharmacol Sci 2005;26:311-317.

[2] Uhl GR, Sora I, Wang Z. *The μ opiate receptor as a candidate gene for pain: polymorphisms, variations in expression, nociception, and opiate responses*. Proc Natl Acad Sci U S A 1999;96:7752-7755.

[3] Sora I, Takahashi N, Funada M, Ujike H, Revay RS, Donovan DM, Miner LL, Uhl GR. *Opiate receptor knockout mice define μ receptor roles in endogenous nociceptive responses and morphine-induced analgesia.* Proc Natl Acad Sci U S A 1997;94:1544-1549.

[4] Bruehl S, Chung OY, Donahue BS, Burns JW. *Anger regulation style, postoperative pain, and relationship to the A118G mu opioid receptor gene polymorphism: a preliminary study.* J Behav Med 2006;29:161-169.

[5] Chou WY, Wang CH, Liu PH, Liu CC, Tseng CC, Jawan B. *Human opioid receptor A118G polymorphism affects intravenous patient-controlled analgesia morphine consumption after total abdominal hysterectomy.* Anesthesiology 2006;105:334-337.

[6] Chou WY, Yang LC, Lu HF, Ko JY, Wang CH, Lin SH, Lee TH, Concejero A, Hsu CJ. *Association of μ-opioid receptor gene polymorphism (A118G) with variations in morphine consumption for analgesia after total knee arthroplasty.* Acta Anaesthesiol Scand 2006;50:787-792.

[7] Coulbault L, Beaussier M, Verstuyft C, Weickmans H, Dubert L, Trégouet D, Descot C, Parc Y, Lienhart A, Jaillon P, Becquemont L. *Environmental and genetic factors associated with morphine response in the postoperative period.* Clin Pharmacol Ther 2006;79:316-324.

[8] Klepstad P, Rakvåg TT, Kaasa S, Holthe M, Dale O, Borchgrevink PC, Baar C, Vikan T, Krokan HE, Skorpen F. *The 118 A > G polymorphism in the human μ-opioid receptor gene may increase morphine requirements in patients with pain caused by malignant disease.* Acta Anaesthesiol Scand 2004;48:1232-1239.

[9] Schinkel AH, Wagenaar E, van Deemter L, Mol CA, Borst P. *Absence of the mdr1a P-glycoprotein in mice affects tissue distribution and pharmacokinetics of dexamethasone, digoxin, and cyclosporine* A. J Clin Invest 1995;96:1698-1705.

[10] Klinck JR, Lindop MJ. *Epidural morphine in the elderly: A controlled trial after upper abdominal surgery.* Anaesthesia 1982;37:907-912.

[11] Hoskin PJ, Hanks GW. *Opioid agonist-antagonist drugs in acute and chronic pain states.* Drugs 1991;41:326-344.

[12] Buchanan WW, Kassam YB. *European experience with flurbiprofen: a new analgesic/anti-inflammatory agent.* Am J Med 1986;80:145-152.

[13] Sunshine S, Olson NZ. *Nonnarcotic analgesics.* In: Wall PD, Melzack R (ed) Textbook of Pain, 3rd edn. Churchill Livingstone, Edinburgh, 1994, pp. 923-942.

[14] Basar H, Yilmaz E, Ozcan S, Buyukkocak U, Sari F, Apan A, Batislam E. *Four analgesic techniques for shockwave lithotripsy: eutectic mixture local anesthetic is a good alternative.* J Endourol 2003;17:3-6.

[15] Ozcan S, Yilmaz E, Buyukkocak U, Basar H, Apan A. *Comparison of three analgesics for extracorporeal shock wave lithotripsy.* Scand J Urol Nephrol 2002;36:281-285.

[16] Pathak KS, Brown RH, Nash CL Jr, Cascorbi HF. *Continuous opioid infusion for scoliosis fusion surgery.* Anesth Analg 1983;62:841-845.

[17] Faul F, Erdfelder E, Lang AG, Buchner A. *G*Power 3: a flexible statistical power analysis program for the social, behavioral, and biomedical sciences.* Behav Res Methods 2007:39:175-191.

[18] Sai K, Kaniwa N, Itoda M, Saito Y, Hasegawa R, Komamura K, Ueno K, Kamakura S, Kitakaze M, Shirao K, Minami H, Ohtsu A, Yoshida T, Saijo N, Kitamura Y, Kamatani N, Ozawa S, Sawada J. *Haplotype analysis of ABCB1/MDR1 blocks in a Japanese population reveals genotype-dependent renal clearance of irinotecan.* Pharmacogenetics 2003;13:741-757.

[19] Cohen J. *Statistical Power Analysis for the Behavioral Sciences (revised edition).* Academic Press, New York, 1977.

[20] Levran O, O'Hara K, Peles E, Li D, Barral S, Ray B, Borg L, Ott J, Adelson M, Kreek MJ. *ABCB1 (MDR1) genetic variants are associated with methadone doses required for effective treatment of heroin dependence.* Hum Mol Genet 2008;17:2219-2227.

In: Opioids: Pharmacology, Clinical Uses and Adverse Effects ISBN 978-1-61942-101-1
Editors: Djavakhi Tvildiani and Kakha Gegechkori

Chapter 8

COGNITIVE-BEHAVIORAL INDICATORS OF ALCOHOLISM PHENOTYPES IN PATIENTS IN OPIOID MAINTENANCE TREATMENT: AN EMPIRICAL ANALYSIS

Samuel Pombo, Filipe Barbosa, Marco Torrado and Nuno Felix da Costa
Nuno Felix da Costa, University of Lisbon, Portugal

ABSTRACT

Polydrug use is common among patients in opioid maintenance programs. Heroin users often abuse alcohol, which may deteriorate the outcome of opioid maintenance treatment.

Excessive alcohol consumption among opioid maintenance patients has been associated with quality of life impairments and with serious social and health costs. Patients who are dependent both on illicit drugs and alcohol may have a poorer treatment outcome than patients without alcohol problems. The clinical and psychosocial treatment of these patients presents challenging work for the clinician. Therefore, treatment outcomes may be further improved if clinical subtypes of substance abusers could be identified and matched to an adequate treatment program.

In this study we aim to assess the prevalence of a drinking problem and analyze the cognitive and behavioral features of problematic alcohol use in opioid addicts according to Cloninger and Lesch's alcoholism typologies in a sample of 102 heroin-dependent patients in Opioid Maintenance Treatment. This sample was selected in the Addiction Unit of the Psychiatric Service of Santa Maria University Hospital, in Lisbon-Portugal.

Results show that alcohol use and alcohol-related problems are frequent among heroin-dependent patients. Study clinical descriptors discriminate Cloninger's type I and type II drinking problem and confirm this binary alcoholism classification in this population. Heroin-dependent patients classified as Cloninger´s type II problem drinkers showed a more severe cognitive-behavior profile than those with a type I alcohol problem, concerning alcohol-taking situation prototypes, beliefs and expectancies about alcohol effects. Data only allows preliminary results about the Lesch's alcoholism classification

This cognitive and behavioral multidimensional assessment has relevant indicators to diagnose different drinking problems among the opioid maintenance programs population. It may improve intervention and treatment outcomes, reducing current health and psychosocial damage associated with an alcohol-abusing lifestyle.

Keywords: Cognitive-behavioral; alcoholism; phenotypes; opioid maintenance treatment.

Opioid Maintenance Treatment (OMT) with methadone or buprenorphine is a broadly used form of substitute therapy, with effective results in heroin dependence trials (West et al., 2000; Stein et al., 2005; Soyka et al. 2008; Costa et al., 2008). Studies demonstrate that it retains patients in treatment, decreases heroin use and related crime and health problems (Bertschy, 1995; Mattick et al., 2003). Even so, in some cases treatment discharge is a common reality. Treatment discontinuation or dropouts seems to be associated with loss of contact with treatment services, non-compliance with program rules, death or other medical problems, transfer to another program and achievement of goals (Magura et al., 1998). In order to improve retention and to identify risk or dropout, treatment enhancement efforts should focus on patient motivation, therapeutic involvement and frequency of session attendance, and also on the therapist perceptions (Simpson et al., 1997). According to our experience, the attendance at a weekly psychotherapeutic group could help to sustain different emotional problems habitually associated with motivation to change, dropout or relapse.

Treating OMT patients with combined heroin, cocaine and alcohol problems is more challenging than working with clients with less opioid polydrug use (Rowan-Szal et al., 2000).

The aim of the study is to (1) screen problematic alcohol use in opiate addicts in maintenance treatment; (2) assess cognitive-behavioral key constructs of drinking such as craving, alcohol related beliefs and expectancies and high-risk situations; (3) measure how alcoholism typologies behave in opiate addicts with an alcohol problem and (4) assess these previous cognitive-behavioral key constructs of drinking across alcoholism subtypes.

Methods and Measures

The sample comprised 102 heroin-dependent patients, admitted in the Addiction Unit of the Psychiatric Service of Santa Maria University Hospital in Lisbon, Portugal.

During the outpatient therapeutical programme clinical and socio-demographic information was collected with a brief standardized interview. After that, the patients fulfill the Michigan Alcoholism Screening Test (MAST). In the second moment, only patients who score positive in the screening procedure (MAST positive) were eligible for the study. As a result, patients complete the Inventory of Drug Taking Situations adapted for alcohol (IDTS), the Alcohol Related Beliefs and Expectations Questionnaire (ABEQ), the Penn Alcohol Craving Scale (PACS) and the substance abuse and dependence disorders section of the Mini International Neuropsychiatric Interview (MINI). The MINI is a short, structured diagnostic interview for DSM-IV and ICD-10 psychiatric disorders, which takes approximately 15 minutes to administer. Patients were administered with the MINI to assess the presence of lifetime DSM-IV diagnoses of alcohol and drug use disorders.

The Alcohol Personal Beliefs and Expectancies Inventory (APBEI) is self-administered instrument constitute by 61 items, design to evaluate beliefs and expectancies related to alcohol effect. To each belief there are five categories of a possible answer (Likert type), from "I don't agree" to "I completely agree". The APBEI has demonstrated good characteristics of reliability and validity in alcohol user populations. The inventory reaches good psychometric properties with highly intern consistency: correlation coefficient was 0.973 to (Split-half), the Spearman-Brown coefficient was equal to 0.986 and the alpha Cronbach was equal to 0.984. Temporal stability was adequate with a Spearman coefficient of correlation equal to 0.764. Factorial analysis isolate 6 factors, that explain 62.62% of the total variance: (F1) Factor 1: Global Positive Effects and Facilitation of Social Interactions; (F2) Factor 2: Expectancies on Activation and Sexual Pleasure effects; (F3) Factor 3: Composed by items that translate expectancies on Positive Effects in Activity and Humour; (F4) Factor 4: Dimension of the expectancies of alcohol might work as Escape to Negative Emotional States; (F5) Factor 5: Translate expectancies of Sexual Disinhibition; and (F6) Factor 6: Express expectancies on alcohol related to Diminution of Negative Feelings about himself and of Evaluated Anxiety. A global result that corresponds to the total of all answers is also obtained This tool may be useful in several contexts, like in clinical practice with alcoholics or individuals with drinking problems, since it allows the operationalization of cognitive variables that are considered to influence behavior decisions as drinking (Gouveia et al., 1993).

Alcohol craving is considered one of the core components of the cognitive-behavioral model of alcoholism and a strong predictor of relapse. Craving was assessed with the PACS (Flannery et al., 1999). This instrument is a 5-item self-administered scale designed to assess the alcohol craving severity (frequency, intensity, duration, resistance, and overall craving) during the previous week. In an alcoholic Portuguese outpatient population, the PACS have revealed good psychometric qualities (Pombo et al., *in press*).

Quantity-Frequency (QF) method was used in order to estimate the average number of drinking days over a certain period (typical week) and then to estimate the average number of drinks consumed per drinking day. The QF drinking variable was then calculated as the product result of those measures (in standard drinks) - average number of drinks per week. A standard drink was defined as one beer, one glass of wine, one glass or shot of liquor.

All subjects were evaluated in a face-to-face interview and asked directly about the items that comprise the operationalized criteria described by each alcoholism typology. Here we provide an overview of the clinical criteria and decision process for subtyping the Cloninger approach and the Lesch alcoholic typology. Patients subtype allocation for Cloninger et al. (1981) model follows the von Knorring et al. (1985) criteria. For type I were the presences of subjective drinking problems start after age 25, first treatment contact after age 30 and few social complications (legal, work problems). Type II included subjective drinking problems start before age 25, first treatment contact before age 30 and frequent social complications (legal, work problems). Decision procedure in the set was: when the specified criteria of each subtype (I or II) was present, subjects received a positive score in each item endorsed (+1), and, when the specified criteria was not in attendance, subjects received a negative score (-1). Afterwards, for patient's allocation purposes, algebraic sum of the items are performed and the quantitative scores were transformed into categorical data on the basis of higher total positive scores (or less negative) in each subtype. Sums equal to 0 were considered to be undiagnosed classification.

The classification procedure of the 4 alcoholism sub-types of Lesch et al. (1988) was based in a computerized Decision Tree. This PC-guided version of patient's allocation (Decision Tree) is nowadays available in computer software in most European languages, including Portuguese, and it has already been used in various international trials (Lesch et al., 2001; Hillmacher et al., 2006; Walter et al., 2006; Pombo et al., 2007; 2009). The descriptors for each type are as follow: Type I: social drinking develops to habitual drinking, medium abstinence syndrome occurs early, craving, positive family history for alcoholism and minimal social effects; Type II: alcohol consumption as a coping strategy against anxiety, suicidal intentions (mainly under the influence of alcohol) and no severe somatic alcohol related disorders or withdrawal; Type III: alcohol consumption as a form of self treatment (depression, sleep disorders), suicidal tendencies, psychiatric co-morbidity, aggressive behavior even without alcohol and mild somatic withdrawal; and Type IV: cerebral disturbances or prenatal damage before the termination of brain development, grand mal seizures (not only during withdrawal), enuresis nocturnal, deterioration of individual's psychic, organic and social sphere.

All researchers that performed the subtyping procedure enclose clinical skills to assess addiction patients and scientific knowledge to manage the principles of each classification system.

In order to accurately identify drugs consumption in our sample; all patients were urine tested for the presence of heroin, cocaine and cannabis metabolites. The urine analysis procedure was performed by staff nurses of our Addiction Unit.

All subjects were informed about the study and given the consent for participation.

The exclusion criteria were: presence of serious physical disease, severe psychiatric disorder (schizophrenia and other psychotic disorders, dementia, delirium), state of alcoholic intoxication during assessment and marked cognitive deficit.

Statistical Analysis

Considering normally distributed data (Kolmogorov-Smirnov test) parametric methods were used to calculate numerical relations between data. Chi-square (2-vs-2), student's t test and ANOVA comparisons were used to study the relation between groups. Pearson correlational analysis technique was used to measure the strength of a supposed linear association between the variables. Statistical analysis was performed with Statistical Package for Social Sciences (SPSS-Version 12.0). Statistical significance was defined at $p < 0.05$.

Results

The sample comprised 102 opiate dependent patients, being 79.4% males (N=81) and 20.6% females (N=21). Age varied between 27 and 53 years, with a mean value of 41.5 years (SD = 6.7). Females (mean age =36.8 years) were significantly ($p<0.01$) younger than males (mean age = 42.7 years). The sample was entirely Caucasian (100%). Regarding marital status, 16.6 % were married, 61.8 % were single, and 20.6% were separated. Education ranged between 2 and 15 years, with a mean value of 7.2 years of school attendance

(SD=2.8). Concerning occupational status, 33.3 % were active workers, 8.8 % were already retired and 57.8% were unemployed. No other significant differences (p >0.05) were found between genders and the socio-demographic features.

In what is considered maintenance for the treatment of heroin-dependent outpatients, 58.4% are allocated in the methadone subgroup, with daily mean dosages of 65.1 mg (SD=22.7); and 41.6% are allocated in the buprenorphine group, with daily mean dosages of 7.4 mg (SD=2.4). The patients report a mean of 20.4 (SD=32.0) months of heroin abstinence.

Urine analysis showed that 14.6% of the patients score positive for opiate metabolites, 19.5% score positive for cocaine metabolites, and 52.4% score positive for cannabis metabolites (THC).

Of 102 patients enrolled, 45.1% (N=46) have positive MAST scores (greater than 7), indicating putative alcohol related problems. Socio-demographic characterization of this sample indicates that, 83.7% were males and 16.3% were females; 12.3 % were married, 65.3 % were single, and 22.4% were separated; education level has a mean value of 6.5 years of school attendance; 28.6 % were active workers, 16.3 % were already retired and 55.1% were unemployed. No significant differences (p >0.05) were found between populations with MAST positive and negative cut-point scores.

Concerning clinical characterization of the problematic alcohol use sample, data shows that the average age of drinking onset was 13.7 (SD=7.5), age of alcohol abuse onset was 13.8 (SD=3.6) and the age of alcohol dependence onset was 28.7 years (SD=6.1). Subjects reported an average number of drinks per week (QF) of 72.1 units (SD=62.0).

History of family alcoholism was positive in 47.9% of the cases, being 39.6% with a father or a mother (2.1%) with an alcohol problem and 2.1% with a grandmother or grandfather (12.5%).

Of the total sample, 39.2% had a lifetime diagnosis of alcohol dependence according to the criteria of DSM-IV (MINI diagnostic interview).

After the alcoholism screening, patients were subtyped according to the following classifications sets. The decision tree system of Lesch typology classified the alcohol dependents in the following way: 33.3 % as type II; 40.0 % as type III and 26.7 % as type IV. Dicothomic typology of Cloninger with the operationalized criteria derived from von Knorring et al. showed that 67.4% of individuals were classified as type I and 32.6% as type II. The IDTS eight subscales profile and second order global categories showed the following mean scores: (UE) Unpleasant Emotions (9.8; SD=8.0); (PD) Physical Discomfort (3.2; SD=3.3), (PE) Pleasant Emotions (6.4; SD=4.3); (TC) Testing Personal Control (3.2; SD=3.1), (UT) Urges and Temptations to Use (3.4; SD=3.7); (CO) Conflict with Others (7.8; SD=7.3); (SO) Social Pressure to Use (3.8; SD=3.9); (PT) Pleasant Times with Others (4.6; SD= 4.4); 1. Negative situations (20.9; SD=18.4); 2. Positive situations (10.9; SD=8.8) and 3. Temptation situations (10.5; SD=10.8). Concerning APBEI, the mean scores for the factors are as follow: F1; mean equal to 60.4; SD=26.8; F2; mean equal to 22.3; SD=10.9; F3; mean equal to 32.5; SD=15.8; F4; mean equal to 27.8; SD=17.6; F5; mean equal to 7.1; SD=3.5; and F6; mean equal to 23.7; SD=16.8. The mean total score for the PACS was 5.6 (SD=6.6).

No significant relationships were found between alcohol related variables (MAST, QF, age onset) and maintenance treatment variables such as buprenorphine or methadone daily mean dosages and drug screening in urine analyses.

PACS total score significantly correlate positive with the following subscales of the IDTS: UE (r = 0.30*); PE. (r = 0.44**), CO. (r = 0.40**); SP. (r = 0.45**) and PT. (r =

0.51**). No significant correlations were found between APBEI and the PACS. Significant positive correlations were observed between the MAST total score and the IDTS subscales UE. (r = 0.40 **); UT. (r = 0.37*) and CO. (r = 0.45**). MAST total score also correlate with the factors F2. (r = 0.33*); F4. (r = 0.45**); F6. (r = 0.46**) and total score (r = 0.33*) of the APBEI. No significant correlations were established between the APBEI, PACS and IDTS and socio-demographic features such as age or education level. Several significant positive correlations were found between the APBEI and the IDTS in the heroin-dependent population with concomitant problem drinking. Table 1 shows the matrix correlations between IDTS and the APBEI scores.

Table 1. matrix correlations between IDTS and the APBEI scores

PABEQ	F1	F2	F3	F4	F5	F6	T
IDTS							
UE	.52**	.55**	.61**	.25	.53**	.25	.55**
PD	.38*	.48**	.47**	.18	.46**	.21	.43**
PE	.36**	.52**	.50**	.13	.60**	.40	.40**
TC	.42**	.48**	.44**	.16	.46**	.23	.43**
UT	.55**	.68**	.57**	.52**	.60**	.51**	.67**
CO	.67**	.70**	.74**	.38**	.60**	.31**	.70**
SO	.42**	.64**	.47**	.23	.57**	.23	.48**
PT	.54**	.76**	.60**	.24	.68**	.19	.58**

** p<0.01; * p<0.05.

Taking into account the Cloninger et al., (1981) classification, the statistical comparative procedure disclosed the following results: Heroin-dependent patients classified as type II problem drinkers showed significative (t=-2.6; p<.05) higher scores in MAST (MAST total score equal to 18.1), when comparing to Heroin-dependent patients classified as type I problem drinkers (MAST total score equal to 12.1); Heroin-dependent patients classified as type II problem drinkers, started to abuse and depend on alcohol (t=4.1, t=4.5, respectively; p<.01) earlier (mean ages of 18.3 and 24.0 years, respectively), than Heroin-dependent patients classified as type I problem drinkers (mean ages of 24.6 and 32.6 years, respectively); Heroin-dependent patients classified as type II problem drinkers, reported significative (t=-2.6; p<.05) higher average number of drinks per week (QF equal to 106.7 units), when comparing to Heroin-dependent patients classified as type I problem drinkers (QF equal to 57.1 units).

For IDTS comparisons in type I and type II patients, total scores were used. Hence, heroin-dependent patients classified as type II problem drinkers showed significative higher scores in UE, PD, TC, UT, CO, N and T, when comparing to heroin-dependent patients classified as type I problem drinkers. Table 2 shows the IDTS scores according to Cloninger typology of alcoholism in heroin-dependent patients.

Regarding APBEI comparisons in type I and type II patients, results showed that heroin-dependent patients classified as type II problem drinkers showed significative (p<0.05) higher scores in positive F1; F3 and total score, when comparing to heroin-dependent patients classified as type I problem drinkers. Table 3 shows the APBEI scores according to Cloninger typology of alcoholism in heroin-dependent patients.

No significant differences ($p > 0.05$) were found between Cloninger subtypes and socio-demographic variables or others such as PACS, methadone or buprenorphine dosages, alcoholism family history or drug screening in urine analyses.

Table 2. IDTS score according to Cloninger typology of alcoholism in heroin-dependent patients

Cloninger Set vs. IDTS	Type I X	(SD)	Type II X (SD)	t test	p
UE. unpleasant emotions	7.0	(6.5)	15.6	(7.5) -3.8	0.01
PD. physical discomfort	2.3	(2.8)	4.9	(4.4) -2.1	0.05
PE. pleasant emotions	6.4	(3.2)	6.7	(4.0)	ns
TC. testing personal control	2.4	(2.3)	4.8	(4.6) -2.0	0.05
UT. urges and temptations	2.6	(2.7)	5.2	(4.6) -2.2	0.05
CO. conflict with others	4.4	(5.0)	14.4	(8.4) -4.8	0.01
SO. social pressure to use	3.3	(3.9)	5.0	(5.5)	ns
PT pleasant times with others	4.0	(3.9)	5.8	(5.2)	ns
N. Negative situations	13.8	(12.3)	34.9	(18.8) -.4.3	0.01
P. Positive situations	10.4	(7.4)	12.6	(8.6)	ns
T. Temptation situations	8.4	(7.8)	15.0	(14.1) -1.9	0.05

Table 3. APBEI scores according to Cloninger typology of alcoholism in heroin-dependent patients

	Type I		Type II t test		p	
Cloninger Set vs. APBEI	X	(SD)	X (SD)			
F1.	52.9	(21.8)	75.8	(27.2)	-2.9	0.05
F2.	20.3	(8.3)	26.5	(13.9)		ns
F3.	27.1	(11.1)	42.9	(17.8)	-3.5	0.01
F4.	25.6	(20.2)	32.8	(11.8)		ns
F5.	6.7	(3.4)	8.0	(3.7)		ns
F6.	21.5	(19.5)	28.6	(10.1)		ns
Total score	122.7	(47.4)	172.3	(61.8)	-2.8	0.05

Lesch alcoholism classification in heroin dependent patients did not showed significant differences regarding APBEI, IDST and PACS; whereas we found a marginal statistical difference ($p < 0.06$) related to the subscale CO of IDTS, in what type IV patients showed higher scores (mean equal to 12.5; SD=7.0), when comparing to type II patients (mean equal to 5.3; SD=7.7). We also observe a tendency to report higher scores in APBEI and IDST in type IV and type III patients, when comparing to type II patients, however, none of these differences were significant ($p > 0.05$).

DISCUSSION

Polysubstance use is an unequivocal realism in modern addictions, been the simultaneous use of alcohol in heroin-dependent populations one of the most frequently and problematic behavior, since the alcohol problem often may remain hidden behind a more prominent illegal drug problem. This concern evidently augments when studies reported the considerable lack of treatment for alcohol related problems that occur among patients in opiate maintenance (El-Bassel et al., 1993).

Like in quite a few studies, the frequency of alcohol related problems in opioid addiction populations was high (Backmund et al., 2003; Rittmannsberger et al., 2000; Dobler-Mikola et al., 2005; Hillebrand et al., 2001; Senbanjo et al., 2006; Stenbacka et al., 2007). The alcohol abuse measurement procedure in our heroin-dependent population undergoing OMT, reached a high prevalence of problem drinking, whether this was achieved by a screening method as MAST cut-point score, or according to the diagnostic criteria of DSM-IV (substance abuse section of MINI). Definitely, alcohol use and alcohol-related problems was confirmed to be common among heroin-dependent patients, in what about half of the patients showed indications of problem drinking and approximately one third meet the lifetime diagnosis of alcohol dependence (Maddux and Elliot, 1975; Joseph and Appel, 1985; Ottomanelli, 1999; El-Bassel et al., 1993; Hillebrand et al., 2001; Stenbacka et al., 2007). Several studies highlight the importance of screening alcohol problems in order to prevent the major impact of his recurrent related-problems, especially if heavy drinking continued to remain undetected in the treatment setting. For example, opioid addicted individuals who abused alcohol had a longer arrest history, higher rate of mortality, greater involvement in secondary abuse of other drugs, more severe psychopathology in childhood, a larger prevalence's of antisocial or borderline personality disorders diagnoses, greater global impairment and are at greater risk of drug overdose (Rounsaville et al. 1982; Joseph and Appel, 1985; Roszell et al., 1986; El-Bassel et al., 1993; Chatham et al., 1995; Best et al., 1999). In addition, an alcohol abusing lifestyle could be particularly dangerous to exposure to HIV duo to the influence of alcohol effect. Certainly, patients who consume alcohol and illicit drugs have a higher probability of risk behaviors and subsequent HIV infection (Ottomanelli, 1992). Patients who drink heavily and participate in an OMT may also be at risk of combined Central Nervous System (CNS) depressant pharmacological effects of both substances. For instance, patients could drink to increase the effects of methadone. However, in this study there was no significant correlation between alcohol-related variables and methadone or buprenorphine dosages, which is not consistent with studies stating that MMT patients with associated excessive alcohol use may need higher methadone dosages (Ottomanelli, 1999) and that additional heroin and alcohol use can be reduced by higher methadone dosages (Hartel et al., 1995; Maxwell and Shinderman, 1999).

We also did not find any relationship between the alcohol-related variables and the drug screening in urine analyses, suggesting that alcohol-related problems was not associated with more illicit drug use, a result contrary to others reviews, that reported a positive association between alcohol use and relapse into illicit drugs (Stenbacka et al., 2007). They underlined as well that alcohol dependence can deteriorate the outcome of methadone treatment (Gossop et al., 2006; Ottomanelli, 1999).

It may be put forward that many opiate dependent individuals report the frequent use of alcohol to cope with psychological discomfort related to heroin addiction rehabilitation. Ottomanelli, (1999) points out that alcohol abuse appeared to be more directly related to biological variables (i.e., potentiator of other drugs, relaxant) and to psychological variables (i.e., stimulus to socialization, and psychopathology), which enhanced the conclusion that alcohol abuse by methadone patients is as much a function of the lifestyle of the addicted individual as a biological need to alleviate withdrawal distress.

As in previous studies focused in alcohol dependent populations, the subtype distribution prevalence's have distinguished the predominance of Cloninger's type I patients (2/3 patients), and Lesch's type II and III (Bleich et al. 2004; Carpenter and Hasin, 2001; Hillmacher et al., 2006; Lykouras et al. 1994; Pombo et al., 2007; Pombo and Lesch, 2009). Recently, a closer examination of patients' classification relationship between Lesch et al. subtypes and Cloninger et al. model found a moderate overlap between Lesch et al. type IV and von Knorring et al criteria of Cloninger Type II. The authors mention that these results may be explained by the overlap of some of the operationalized criteria used to define each alcoholic subtype (Pombo and Lesch, 2009).

Approaching the alcoholic subtypes classification on a basis of a spectrum of severity, Cloninger type I and Lesch type II and III should be considered as a moderate severity subgroup and Cloninger type II and Lesch type VI as a high severity subgroup (Pombo and Lesch, 2009).

Craving can be defined as a strong desire/urge towards alcohol consumption. In the study analysis, PACS positively correlated with some subscales of the IDTS, which means that the heroin-dependent population with a drinking problem who reports more alcohol-related craving in the most recent week, tend to generally identify triggers to use alcohol associated with pleasant times with others, social pressure to use, conflict with others, pleasant and unpleasant emotions. These results suggested that alcohol craving is a regular associate of alcohol use emotional triggers. In some extent, these findings go in accordance with previous studies who found that alcohol dependent "cravers" showed significantly higher scores in negative emotions (Rubonis et al., 1994; Cooney et al., 1997; Litt et al., 2000; Andersohn and Kiefer; 2004) as depression, anxiety or aggressivity, supporting the concept of negative and positive craving - cognitive component of craving induced by negative and positive emotions (Pombo et al., *in press*). Contrary to expected, the PACS did not correlate with the Urges and Temptations to Use subscale of IDTS.

Concerning the Cloninger et al., (1981) classification, heroin-dependent patients classified as type II problem drinkers showed more alcohol-related problems, started to abuse and depend on alcohol earlier and reported higher average number of drinks per week, when comparing to heroin-dependent patients classified as type I problem drinkers. These results from the clinical profile of the sample clearly discriminate the type I and type II Cloninger's *et al.* (1981) approach and visibly validate this binary alcoholism classification in an opioid addiction population with concomitant alcohol abuse problem. According to this classification, type I patients, recognized as low-severity/vulnerability subgroup, are characterized by showing a later onset of the drinking problem and less alcohol related problems, and type II patients, acknowledged as high-severity/vulnerability subgroup, by an early onset of the drinking problem, family history of alcoholism problems, antecedents of psychopathology and severe alcohol related problems (Babor and Caetano, 2006).

Back in 1985, Marlatt and Gordon developed an empirical eight-category of excessive drinking situations based on the circumstances that surround the after-treatment relapse episode of the alcoholics. Comprehensive evaluations of relapse situations have been demonstrating negative situation triggers with a fundamental role in the alcohol consume (type II re)engagement. For example, the study of Marlatt and Gordon (1985) concluded that in 35% of the cases the relapses occur by triggers related to negative emotions, 16% interpersonal conflicts with others and 20% by social pressure. Another study concluded that 62–73% of relapse episodes are related to negative emotions and social pressure (Lowman et al., 1996). On the grounds of this work, cognitive and behavioral relapse prevention programs for the psychological treatment of addictions focus on training clients in identifying and coping with their own high-risk situations for heavy drinking. This intervention might be assist with the fulfillment of a psychometric tool as the IDTS that offers a broad profile of the situations in which a client has used alcohol in the past year. Certainly, according to Turner et al., (1997), the implementation of IDTS as a treatment planning tool in clinical practice offers the therapist an effortlessly administered aid to the detection of a patient's high-risk situations for use of a particular drug.

One of the main aims of this research was to assess how the cognitive-behavioral taxonomy of excessive drinking situations could respond to the dichotomic classification of alcohol abuse of Cloninger. So, when considering alcohol use triggers assessed by the scores of IDTS taxonomy, results showed that heroin-dependent patients classified as type II problem drinkers were significantly more likely to abuse on alcohol in situations related to UE, PD, TC, UT, CO, N and T, than those classified as heroin-dependent patients classified as type I problem drinkers. In general, heroin-dependent patients classified as type II problem drinkers reported a more severe alcohol-taking profile than those with type I alcohol problem. This fact goes in conformity with previous studies that found that high negative profile patients have elevated alcohol dependence scores (Annis and Graham, 1995; Turner et al., 1997). Nevertheless, with further examination we could observe that heroin-dependent patients classified as type II problem drinkers were much more vulnerable to negative situation triggers like intrapsychic unpleasant emotions (e.g. anger, anxiety, depression) or interpersonal conflituality (e.g.., discussions with others), than heroin-dependent patients classified as type I problem drinkers. These results are consistent with Waldrop et al., (2007), who compared high-risk triggers and situations among persons with alcohol dependence or cocaine dependence, with or without posttraumatic stress disorder (PTSD). The authors observe that individuals with PTSD+ reported significantly greater substance use in response to negative situations, as compared to PTSD− individuals, supporting this finding with the self-medication theory, in which subjects who experience high rates of negative situations use substances in an attempt to minimize such symptoms. In line with this construction, that enhances the negative reward properties of alcohol, our current findings regarding alcohol use situational triggers and the Cloninger typology might be explain by the high severity profile of disease that typically characterized type II patients, notable by an early onset and frequent psychiatric comorbidity (Babor and Caetano, 2006; Pombo and Lesch, 2009).

These two different IDTS profiles identified from type I/II patients may prove to be suitable for research analysis, but also of greater relevance for clinical intervention within a cognitive-behavioral perspective. Indeed, from a cognitive and behavioral psychological standpoint, we may suggest the development of intervention strategies designed to increase patient's coping self-efficacy, in order to improve perceived internal control over alcohol use. This proposal should have particular focus in type II individuals, since they present a higher severity profile, particular vulnerable to negative situation triggers (e.g. anxiety, social pressure) and research indicates that the greater the level of alcohol dependence, the lower the confidence in the ability to resist the urge to drink heavily in high-risk situations, especially in situations involving unpleasant emotions and conflict with others (Sklar et al., 1997). For these patients, programmes that encourage stress management and social skills training may be essential. In the future we should afford empirical support for the hypothesis that type II patients present a lack of perceived control over alcohol use and a lower confidence in the ability to resist drinking heavily in high-risk situations.

Expectancies usually result form the drinker previous direct and indirect learning experiences with alcohol, and are presumed to be central in decisions to drink (Connors et al., 1988). Generally, drinkers were able to identify quite a few areas of alcohol effects. For example, reduction of negative emotional states, global positive effect, sexual activation, tension reduction, social anxiety reduction, or decreased loneliness and boredom. Almost certainly, drinkers may be more susceptible to use alcohol if they enclose the belief that the alcohol ingestion is an efficient way of dealing with the own negative emotions and facilitate a more affirmative social behavior. All these expectancies are thought to operate in decision making processes and are hypothesized to have a prevailing independently effect on drinking behaviors. A broad evaluation of personal expectancies about the alcohol effect provides to the clinician a better understanding of the cognitive dimension of patient's decisions to drink and also allows a more accurate elaboration of therapeutic programs, mostly in populations with polysubstance use. In methadone maintenance patients, alcohol is predominantly used to fulfill specific functions as helping to relax; stop feeling bored; make yourself feel better when low or depressed; forget problems; help to get to sleep; increase the effects of methadone or any other drug; help to ''get going'' in the morning; stop feeling sick in the morning and calm after using other drugs.

As expected, APBEI discriminate individuals with different levels of problem drinking. Study revealed that heroin-dependent patients classified as type II problem drinkers endorse generally higher levels of alcohol related-expectancies, especially about positive global effects and social interaction facilitation and positive effects on activation and humor, when comparing to heroin-dependent patients classified as type I problem drinkers. This finding goes in accordance with numerous studies, who concluded that individuals who drink more and present a higher problem drinking severity have significantly more positive expectancies about the alcohol effects, which will result in desirable outcomes who promote the increase of alcohol use (Brown et al., 1985; Connors *et al.,* 1988; Stacy et al., 1990; Oei and Baldwin 1994; Brown et al. 1998; Oei et al., 1998; Finn et al. 2000).

Even though, it's important to question why type II patients, acknowledged to exhibit and recognized more alcohol related consequences, report higher levels of expectancies related to the putative alcohol effect when they face up higher levels of negative outcome effects. It seems that the behavioral and social consequences related to alcohol abuse did not influence as much alcohol related cognitions in type II problem drinkers. Self-medication hypothesis might attempt to explain this conception, given the fact that patients who experience more psychological distress, like type II patients (high-severity/vulnerability subgroup), may achieve more reward properties derived from the ability of alcohol play down such negative feelings and symptoms. Other alternative explanation implicates a particular cluster of personality traits that generally characterized type II patients – high novelty seeking and low harm avoidance. These traits reflecting impulsivity and desinhibition may account to a greater exploration of the environment and also make type II patients more vulnerable to pharmacological benefits of alcohol, which could enhance alcohol related cognitions.

These assertions recognized that cognitions could also account to sustain the higher prevalence's of alcohol related problems in type II patients. Indeed, the combination of positive cognitions related to alcohol effect with impulsivity, a poor inhibitory control quality that noticeably characterized Cloninger type II problem drinker's profile, could explain why these patients have difficulties in restrain problematic drinking and present a poorer prognosis.

Cognitions might predict alcohol use in several drinking situations. In fact, expectancies reported by alcohol users more often deal with intrapersonal and interpersonal conflicts in social situations (Connors et al., 1988). As predicted, APBEI positive correlates with IDTS subscales, with the significant coefficients ranging from a low 0.31 (APBEI total score vs. CO subscale of IDTS) to a high 0.74 (APBEI F4 vs. CO subscale of IDTS). These findings clearly suggest that patients who endorse more general positive beliefs and expectancies related to alcohol effect tend to drank heavily across more intra-inter personal situations. We may consider that in high risk-situations for alcohol use, beliefs and expectancies related to alcohol effect become more prominent, rising the vulnerability for drinking behavior. As Connors et al. (1988) mention, "if an adequate coping response is not available or not emitted, there results a decreased sense of self-efficacy and concomitant positive outcome expectancies regarding alcohol, which taken together lead to an increased probability that the alcoholic will drink in that situation". In a study related to drinking outcome expectancies during relapse situations among male alcoholics, the authors reported that almost half of the expectancies reported dealt with drinking as an aid in coping with a social situation, another one-quarter of the expectancies dealt with drinking to gain control of a situation. Interestingly, in a recent report by Blume et al., (2006), it was concluded that cognitions about drinking may not only predict consumption patterns, but also may predict the experience of negative drinking consequences. According to the authors, a significant portion of recent consequences experienced by individuals were not necessarily related to drinking per se, but rather were related to cognitions; for instance, the expected effects of alcohol and the self-efficacy for successfully negotiating high-risk situations without drinking heavily.

Data reduction only allows preliminary results regarding the Lesch alcoholism classification in heroin dependent patients, in what observes a tendency in type IV patients to present a high severity profile regarding the cognitive and behavioral dimensions assessed. This tendency is congruent with a high severity subgroup as Lesch type IV patients (Pombo and Lesch, 2009).

In the study we should consider some limitations: Like in other studies, our data demonstrate a high prevalence of drinking problems among patients undergoing opiate maintenance treatment. However, comparisons across studies should be done cautiously, since diverse study methods have used different instruments to assess alcohol use and abuse, producing some heterogeneity in the results prevalence's. In the study we did not measure other psychological dimensions that could account for the differences in the IDTS profiles. In some extent, other possible explanation accounting for the differences in IDTS profiles between type I and type II patients could be the notion of motivation to change (Prochaska and DiClemente, 1986). Indeed, studies have argued that readiness to change account for the differentiation of IDTS drinking profiles, with more motivated people reporting higher overall IDTS scores or greater differentiation of IDTS subscales and least motivated showing low totals scores and undifferentiated profiles (Annis and Graham; 1995; Turner et al., 1997). As Turner et al. (1997) states, patients with lack of awareness of their drinking (pre-contemplation stage) would have little interest, and maybe little awareness of how their affective states and external circumstances influenced their alcohol use; on the other hand, patients that have made a decision to change (determination stage), would have paid more attention on their alcohol use patterns. Moreover, addiction denial could also provide another plausible interpretation for the differences in IDTS in the subtypes. Alcohol abuse denial defines the notion of the drinker refusal to acknowledge his pathological alcohol use or minimizing the relation between alcohol consumption and his psychological, organic and social problems. In psychodynamic terms, denial is usually considered as an unconscious ego defense mechanism. Other authors propose that alcoholic denial is more related to cognitive failure than an ego defense mechanism, consisting in a diminished capacity for insight, for example, due to executive function failure (Rinn et al., 2002). A recent study performed in alcoholic patients have demonstrated that Cloninger's type II patients reported lower levels of alcoholism denial, when compared with type I patients (Pombo et al., 2008a). Indeed, since type I patients tend to become more defensive regarding alcohol use it will be expected that they tend to refuse or turn hesitant in identifying their real high-risk situations, and as result, a lower and more undifferentiated IDTS profile could emerge. In the psychometric study of IDTS performed by Turner et al., (1997), other dimensions were found to influence IDTS scores. For example, the authors concluded that individuals who reported that they spend little time using unaccompanied and experience pressure from family or friends to use substances, had higher scores on the IDTS interpersonal subscales of PT and SP, while individuals who assumed spending more time using substances alone had elevations on the IDTS intrapersonal subscales of UE and PD.

We also may found some inconsistencies regarding the alcohol related expectancies in this population, since this association may vary by population heterogeneity, polysubstance use and levels and time-course of substance use.

The screening for drug metabolites in urine analyses, a procedure that incorporates the clinical routine of our addiction unit, was properly controlled by the nurse staff. Nevertheless, alcohol use was only assessed by patients self-reports providing a possible reliability limitation in the interview, given the fact that participants with an excessive alcohol use may tend to underestimate or deny alcohol consumption and related problems. Therefore, a more accurate determination of patient alcohol consumption levels, for example, urine analyses or liver function, should be performed. For example, Stenbacka et al., (2007), posits that most studies on MMT patients consider the alcohol use information based on records from interviews and questionnaires, and only occasionally using laboratory tests. Indeed, a recent study of the authors found a significant association between the number of alcohol-related diagnoses prior to treatment and a positive 5HTOL/5HIAA (sensitive biomarker of acute alcohol consumption) test during MMT.

It's also important to bring up some technical issues applying the Lesch classification procedure to opiate dependent patients who meet also the criteria for alcohol dependence, since items related to alcohol withdrawal or seizures could also be attached to a frequent behavior in this population like higher levels of benzodiazepine use.

Finally, we should also consider limitations due to the relatively small sample size of the study, the heterogeneity of the population and the fact that gender differences were not examined due to small cell sizes. So, it's not clear without further evaluation that these data could be generalized to other populations of drinkers.

Conclusion

A range of different factors that differ from person to person influences aetiology and outcomes of addiction. In research and clinical practice, the evaluation of different functions such as screening, assessment, diagnosis, treatment planning and follow-up, are an essential step to identify behaviors and associated problems and to improve prevention and treatment in a population that often seeks help related to the misuse of substances (Hester and Miller, 2003).

Studies have been assembling empirical evidence for the treatment of alcohol dependence in general (Johnson and Ait-Daoud, 2000; Hester and Miller, 2003; Saitz, 2007), particularly relapse prevention pharmaceutical agents such as naltrexone and acamprosate. In the meantime, when we extend the clinical management of an alcohol problem to methadone-using patients, we may face several boundaries in the treatment outcome, mostly related to the complexity inherent to polysubstance use, abuse or dependence and also because we must consider the exception of a pharmacologically effective tool in the treatment of alcoholism such as naltrexone since it is contraindicated in methadone-using patients.

A more accurate clinical establishment of the nature of the relationship between alcohol and opioids, would be useful in planning treatment for opioid dependent patients with concurrent alcohol use, with particular focus on relapse prevention not only for heroin use but for other drugs and alcohol as well (Stenbacka et al., 2007; Srivastava et al., 2008).

The study concluded that in general, heroin-dependent patients classified as type II problem drinkers demonstrate a more severe alcohol-taking profile than those with a type I alcohol problem. Nevertheless, upon closer examination we were be able to identify different situation-specific prototypes of alcohol use, in which heroin-dependent patients classified as type II problem drinkers were much more vulnerable to negative situation triggers like intrapsychic unpleasant emotions or interpersonal confliction, than heroin-dependent patients classified as type I problem drinkers. These high-risk situations in type II patients, along with more positive beliefs and expectancies about alcohol effect may increase the chance for ineffective coping responses with an unremitting alcohol abuse pattern. Therefore, these cognitive-behavioral indicators should help the clinician to better tailor the intervention in this particular population. Indeed, treatment outcomes may be further improved if clinical subtypes of substance abusers could be identified and matched to an adequate treatment. Given this potential impact, evidence comes from the observation that type A alcoholics have better outcomes in interactional treatment and do more poorly with coping skills training and in opposition, type B alcoholics had better outcomes with the coping skills treatment and worse outcomes with interactional therapy (Litt et al., 1992). To some extent, these findings from Litt et al. (1992) may have clinical implications in our study, since type A patients from Babor et al. (1992) and type I from Cloninger et al. (1981) are in some way similar (low-severity/vulnerability subgroup), as Babor et al. (1992) type B and Cloninger et al. (1981) type II (high-severity/vulnerability subgroup).

With a cognitive-behavioral multidimensional assessment of relevant indicators such as alcohol craving, type and degree of beliefs and expectations related to alcohol effects and the identification of taxonomic high-risk situations for alcohol use would enable the substance abuse psychological health-care to focus on the management of specific areas to prevent problem drinking and reduce current harm associated with their lifestyle. Indeed, the cognitive-behavioral measurement and conceptualization underlying the pathological drinking in heroin dependence is essential in the development of successful psychoeducational messages and relapse prevention strategies related to alcohol use. Cognitive-behavioral therapists should teach patients a broad range of coping skills to avoid or deal with the return of previous excessive alcohol use, such as problem solving, challenging distorted thoughts, relaxation, assertiveness, modeling and functional analysis. In cases following an assessment of specific alcohol-use functions reported by patients with polysubstance use pattern, the mental health clinicians, in interaction with patients, should encourage them to indentify high-risk situations in as much detail as possible and develop alternative ways of fulfilling these functions. Nevertheless, it is imperative to posit that these psychological strategies only succeed with patients if therapists always keep up efforts to build a good therapeutic relationship with them. For example, Dundon et al., (2008), focused on a factor that is common to all types of psychosocial treatments for substance abuse—the therapeutic alliance between the patient and the clinician. According to the authors, the therapeutic alliance reflects the nature and strength of the affective bond between patient and primary clinician in their collaboration in identifying and working toward the patient's treatment goals.

Future investigations need to be considered in order to continuously update the cognitive-behavioral background with new empirical findings about clinical subgroups and polysubstance abuse life courses.

References

Agrawal, S., Sobell, M. B., & Sobell, L. C. (2007). The Timeline Followback: A scientifically and clinically useful tool for assessing substance use. In R. F. Belli, F. P. Stafford, & D. F. Alwin (Eds.), *Using calendar and diary methodologies in life events research.* Beverly Hills, CA: Sage Publications.

Allen, J. P. and Wilson, V. B. (2003) *Assessing alcohol problems: A guide for clinicians and researchers.* National Institute of Alcohol Abuse and Alcoholism, Bethesda.

Almog YJ, Anglin MD, Fisher DG. (1993) Alcohol and heroin use patterns of narcotics addicts: gender and ethnic differences. *Am. J. Drug Alcohol Abuse;* 19:219–38.

Amaro H, Mangual S, Nieves RL.(2004a) Spirituality in recovery: *An educational group curriculum for women in recovery.* Boston Consortium of Services for Families in Recovery, Public Health Commission, Boston, MA.

Amaro H, Nieves RL, Saunders L. (2004b) Women's Leadership Training Institute: *An educational group curriculum for women in recovery.* Boston Consortium of Services for Families in Recovery, Public Health Commission, Boston, MA.

Ambrose ML, Bowden SC, Whelan G (2001). Working memory impairments in alcohol-dependent participants without clinical amnesia. *Alcoholism: Clinical and Experimental Research;* vol.25, No.2, pp 185-191.

Andersohn, F. & Kiefer, F. (2004). Depressive mood and craving during alcohol withdrawal: association and interaction. *German Journal Psychiatry,* 7, 6-11.

Anglin, M. D., Almog, I. J., Fisher, D. G., & Peters, K. R. (1989). Alcohol use by heroin addicts: Evidence for an inverse relationship. A study of methadone maintenance and drug-free treatment samples. *American Journal of Drug and Alcohol Abuse*. 15, 191–207.

Annis, H.M. & Martin, G. (1985). Inventory of Drug-Taking Situations. Toronto, Canada: Addiction Research Foundation.

Annis, H. M., & Graham, J. M. (1995). Profile types on the Inventory of Drinking Situations: Implications for relapse prevention counselling. *Psychology of Addictive Behaviours*. 9, 176-182.

Arasteh, K., Des Jarlais, D.C., Perlis, T. (2008). Alcohol and HIV sexual risk behaviors among injection drug users. *Drug Alcohol Depend*. 95, 54–61.

Avants SK, Warburton LA, Margolin A. (2001) Spiritual and religious support in recovery from addiction among HIV-positive injection drug users. *Journal of Psychoactive Drugs;* 33(1): 39–46.

Babor, T.F., Biddle-Higgins, J.C., Saunders, J.B. & Monteiro, M.G. (2001). AUDIT: The Alcohol Use Disorders Identification Test: Guidelines for Use in Primary Health Care. Geneva, Switzerland: World Health Organization.

Babor, T. F., De Hofmann, M. I., Boca, F. K., Hesselbrock, V., Meyer, R. E., Dolinsky, Z. S. & Rounsaville, B. (1992) Types of alcoholics, I: evidence for an empirically derived typology based on indicator of vulnerability and severity. *Archives of General Psychiatry*. 49, 599-608.

Babor & Caetano (2006) Subtypes of substance dependence and abuse: implications for diagnostic classification and empirical research. *Addiction*. 101(sup):104-110.

Backmund M, Schutz CG, Meyer K, Eichenlaub D, Soyka M. (2003) Alcohol consumption in heroin users, methadone-substituted and codeine-substituted patients-frequency and correlates of use. *Eur. Addict. Res;* 9:45–50.

Baetz M, Bowen R, Jones G, Koru-Sengul T.(2006) How spiritual values and worship attendance relate to psychiatric disorders in the Canadian population. *Canadian Journal of Psychiatry;* (51): 654–661.

Bandura, A. (1977) Self-efficacy: toward a unifying theory of behavioural change. *Psychological Review*. 84, 191–215.

Ball S. A. Carroll K. M. ; Babor T. F ; Rounsaville B. (1995) Subtypes of cocaine abusers: support for a Type A-Type B distinction. *Journal of Consulting and Clinical Psychology*. 63, 115-124.

Barrett ME, Simpson D, Lehman WE.(1988) Behavioral changes of adolescents in drug abuse intervention programs. *Journal of Clinical Psychology;* 44: 461–473.

Bartzokis G, Beckson M, Lu PH et al. Age-related brain volume reductions in amphetamine and cocaine addicts and normal controls: implications for addiction research. *Psychiatry Res*. 2000; 98:93_102.

Beck A, Wright F, Newman C, Liesh B. (1993) *Cognitive Therapy of Substance Abuse*. New York: Guilford Press.

Bellis, M., Hughes, K., Bennett, A. and Thomson, R. (2003), 'The role of an international nightlife resort in the proliferation of recreational drugs', *Addiction,* 98, pp. 1713–21.

Bergeret J. (1983) Toxicomania e personalidade, Rio de Janeiro, Zahar Ed.

Bertschy, G. (1995). Methadone maintenance treatment: An update. *European Archives of Psychiatry and Clinical Neuroscience*. 245, 114–125.

Best, D., Gossop, M., Lehmann, P., Harris, J., & Strang, J. (1999). The relationship between overdose and alcohol consumption among methadone maintenance patients. *Journal of Substance Use*. 4, 41– 44.

Beswick, T., Best, D., Rees, S., Coomber, R., Gossop, M., Strang, J., (2001). Multiple drug use: patterns and practices of heroin and crack use in a population of opiate addicts in treatment. *Drug Alcohol. Rev*. 20, 201–204.

Bleich S, Bayerlein K, Reulbach U, Hillemacher T, Bönsch D, Mugele B, Kornhuber J, Sperling W. (2004) Homocysteine levels in patients classified according to Lesch's typology. *Alcohol and Alcoholism*. 39(6), 493-498.

Blume AW, Lostutter T, Schmaling K, Marlatt A. (2003) Beliefs about drinking behavior predict drinking consequences, *Journal of Psychoactive Drugs*. 35(3), 395–399.

Blum RW, Halcón L, Beuhring T, Pate E, Campell-Forrester S, Venema A. (2003) Adolescent health in the Caribbean: risk and protective factors. *American Journal of Public Health;* 93(3): 456–460.

Booth B, Leukefeld C, Falck R, Wang J, Carlson R, (2006). Correlates of rural methamphetamine and cocaine users: results from a multistate community study. *J. Stud. Alcohol*. 67, 493–501.

Bolla KI, Ernst M, Kiehl KA, Mouratidis M, Eldreth DA et al (2004) Prefrontal cortical dysfunction in abstinent cocaine abusers. *J. Neuropsych. Clin*. N 16:456–464.

Bolla KI, Rothman R, Cadet JL. Dose-related neurobehavioral effects of chronic cocaine use. *J. Neuropsychiatry Clin. Neurosci*. 1999; 11:361_369.

Bovasso, G., Cacciola, J. (2003). The long-term outcomes of drug use by methadone maintenance patients. *J. Behav. Health Serv. Res*. 30, 290–303.

Boys, A., Fountain, J., Marsden, J. et al. (1999), 'What influences young people's use of drugs? *A qualitative study of decision-making', Drugs: Education, Prevention and Policy*. 6, pp. 373–89.

Breslin, F. C., Sobell, L. C., Sobell, M. B., & Agrawal, S. (2000). A comparison of a brief and long version of the Situational Confidence Questionnaire. *Behaviour Research and Therapy*. 38, 1211-1220

Brewer DD, Catalano RF, Haggerty K, Gainey RR, Fleming CB.(1998) A meta-analysis of predictors of continued drug use during and after treatment for opiate addiction. *Addiction;* 93: 73–92.

Brown, S. A., Goldman, M. S., Inn, A. et al. (1980) Expectations of reinforcement from alcohol: Their domain and relation to drinking patterns. *Journal of Consulting and Clinical Psychology*. 48, 419–426.

Brown SA, Christiansen BA, Goldman MS (1987). The Alcohol Expectancy Questionnaire: an instrument for the assessment of adolescent and adult alcohol expectancies. *J. Stud. Alcohol*. Sep; 48(5):483-91.

Brown SA, Goldman MS, Christiansen BA. (1985) Do alcohol expectancies mediate drinking patterns of adults? *Journal of Consulting and Clinical Psychology*. 53, 512-19.

Brown SA, Carrello PD, Vik PW, Porter RJ. (1998) Change in alcohol effect and self-efficacy expectancies during addiction treatment. *Substance Abuse;* 19:155–67.

Brown BS, O'Grady KE, Farrell EV, Fechner IS, Nurco DN.(2001) Factors associated with frequency of 12-step attendance by drug abuse clients. *American Journal of Drug and Alcohol Abuse;* 27: 147–160.

Byqvist, S., (2006). Patterns of drug use among drug misusers in Sweden gender differences. *Subst. Use Misuse.* 41, 1817–1835.

Caputo F, Addolorato G, Domenicali M,_Mosti A, Viaggi M, Trevisani F, Gasbarrini G, Bernardi M and Stefanini G , & The Services For Addiction Treatment (2002) Short-term methadone administration reduces alcohol consumption in non-alcoholic heroin addicts. *Alcohol Alcohol.* 37, 164 –16 8.

Cardoso, J.M., Barbosa, A., Ismail, F. and Pombo, S. (2006) Neter Alcoholic Typology (NAT). *Alcohol and Alcoholism.* 41, 133-139.

Carpenter KM, Hasin DS (2001) Reliability and discriminant validity of the type I/II and type A/B alcoholic subtype classifications in untreated problem drinkers: a test of the Apollonian-Dionysian hypothesis. *Drug and Alcohol Dependence.* 63, 51-67.

Chatham, L. R., Rowan-Szal, G. A., Joe, G. W., Brown, B. S., & Simpson, D. D. (1995). Heavy drinking in a population of methadone-maintained clients. *Journal of Studies on Alcohol.* 7, 417– 422.

Ciccocioppo R., Antonelli L., Biondini M., Perfumi M., Pompei P., Massi M. (2002) Memory impairment following combined exposure to delta(9)-tetrahydrocannabinol and ethanol in rats. *European Journal of Pharmacology;* 449:245-251.

Cooney, N.L., Litt, M.D., Morse, P.A., Bauer, L.O. & Gaupp, L. (1997). Alcohol cue reactivity, negative mood reactivity, and relapse in treated alcoholics men. *Journal Abnormal Psychology.* 106, 243-250.

Connors G J; O'Farrell T J; Pelcovits M A. (1988). Drinking outcome expectancies among male alcoholics during relapse situations. *British journal of addiction.* 83(5), 561-6.

Colzato L, Huizinga M & B Hommel. (2009) Recreational cocaine polydrug use impairs cognitive flexibility but not working memory. *Psychopharmacology;* 207:225–234.

Costa NF, Pombo S, Barbosa F. (2008) A propósito da avaliação clínica numa consulta de toxicodependências *Toxicodependências.* 14, 25-34.

Cloninger, C. R., Bohman, M. & Sigvardsson, S (1981). Inheritance alcohol abuse: cross fostering analysis of adopted men. *Archives of General Psychiatry.* 38, 861868.

Cunningham JA. (2000) Remissions from drug dependence: Is treatment a prerequisite? *Drug and Alcohol Dependence;* 59: 211−213.

D'Aunno, T., & Vaughn, T. E. (1992). Variations in methadone treatment practices. Results from a national study. *Journal of the American Medical Association.* 267, 253– 258.

Dafters R, Hoshi R, Talbot A (2004). Contribution of cannabis and MDMA ("ecstasy") to cognitive changes in long-term polydrug users. *Psychopharmacology;* 173:405–410.

Darke, S., Ross, J., Teesson, M. (2007). The Australian Treatment Outcome Study ATOS: what have we learnt about treatment for heroin dependence? Drug Alcohol. Rev. 26, 49–54.

Darke S, Sims J, McDonald S, Wickes W (2000) Cognitive impairment among methadone maintenance patients. *Addiction;* 95:687, 695.

Dawes MA, Antelman SM, Vanyukov MM, Giancola P, Tarter RE, Susman EJ, et al.(2000) Developmental sources of variation in liability to adolescent substance use disorders. *Drug and Alcohol Dependence;* 61(1): 3–14.

Demir B, Ulug B, Lay E, Erbas B (2002). Regional cerebral blood flow and neuropsychological functioning in early and late onset alcoholism. *Psychiatric Research;* 1:115(3):115-25.

Dermatis H, Guschwan MT, Galanter M, Bunt G. (2004) Orientation toward spirituality and self-help approaches in the therapeutic community. *Journal of Addictive Diseases;* 23(1).

Dobler-Mikola, A., Hattenschwiler, J., Meili, D., Beck, T., Boni, E., Modestin, J. (2005). Patterns of heroin, cocaine, and alcohol abuse during long-term methadone maintenance treatment. *J. Subst. Abuse Treat.* 29, 259–265.

Downey, K., Helmus, T., Schuster, C. (2000). Treatment of heroin-dependent poly-drug abusers with contingency management and buprenorphine maintenance. *Exp. Clin. Psychopharmacol.* 8, 176–184.

DiClemente, C.C. & Hughes, S.O. (1990). Stages of change profiles in alcoholism treatment. *Journal of Substance Abuse,* 2, 217-235.

Dundon W, Pettinati H, Lynch K, Xie H, Varillo K, Makadon C, Oslin D. (2008) The therapeutic alliance in medical-based interventions impatcs outcome in treating alcohol dependence. *Drug and Alcohol Dependence* 95, 230–236.

Duka T, Townshend JM, Collier K, Stephens DN (2003) Impairment in cognitive functions after multiple detoxifications in alcoholic inpatients. *Alcoholism: Clinical and Experimental Research;* Vol.27, No10, pp 1563-1572.

Dvorak A, Pombo S, Ismail F, Barbosa A, Cardoso JM, Figueira ML, Walter H, Lesch OM (2006). Tipologias da dependência do álcool e o seu significado para a terapêutica médica. *Acta Psiquiátrica Portuguesa* 52, 1693-1705.

Edwards G, Gross MM (1976). Alcohol dependence: provisional description of a clinical syndrome. *Br. Med. J.* May 1;1058–1061

El-Bassell N, Schilling RF. (1992) 15 month follow-up of women methadone patients taught skills to reduce heterosexual HIV transmission. *Public Health Reports;* 107: 500–504.

El-Bassel, N., Schilling, R. F., Turnbull, J. E., & Su, K.-H. (1993). Correlates of alcohol use among methadone patients. *Alcoholism: Clinical and Experimental Research.* 17, 681–686.

Eldreth DA, Matochik JA, Cadet JL, Bolla KI (2004) Abnormal brain activity in prefrontal brain regions in abstinent marijuana users. *Neuroimage;* 23:914:920.

Ellison CG. (1991) Religious involvement and subjective well-being. *Journal of Health and Social Behavior;* 32(1): 80–99.

EMCDDA (2007), Selected issue, Drugs and driving, European Monitoring Centre for Drugs and Drug Addiction, Lisbon.

EMCDDA (2009), Polydrug use: patterns and responses. European Monitoring Centre for Drugs and Drug Addiction, Lisbon.

Ersche KD, Fletcher PC, Lewis SJ et al. (2005) Abnormal frontal activations related to decision-making in current and former amphetamine and opiate dependent individuals. *Psychopharmacology;* 180:612_623.

Everitt B. (1997) Craving cocaine cues: cognitive neuroscience meets drug addiction research. *Trends Cogn. Sci.* (Regul. Ed.); 1: 1.

Ewing JA (1984) Detecting alcoholism. The CAGE questionnaire. *JAMA;* 252(14):1905-7.

Fairbank, J.A., Dunteman, G.H., & Condelli, W.S. (1993). Do methadone patients substitute other drugs for heroin? Predicting substance use at 1-year follow-up. *American Journal of Drug and Alcohol Abuse.* 19, 465–474.

Fein G, Di Sclafani V, Meyerhoff DJ (2002) Prefrontal cortical volume reduction associated with frontal cortex function deficit in 6-week abstinent crack-cocaine dependent men. *Drug Alcohol Depend*; 68:87:93.

Feng Y, Xun SS, Wang XH. (1999) Study on depression and anxiety of 50 cases heroin reliers before and after detoxification therapy. *Chinese Journal of Drug Abuse Prevention and Treatment;* 18(1): 12-15.

Flannery, B.A., Volpicelli, J.R. & Pettinati. (1999). Psychometric properties of the Penn Alcohol Craving Scale. *Alcoholism: Clinical Experimental Research.* 8, 1289-1295.

Flannery, B., Morgenstern, J., McKay, J., Wechsberg, W., Litten, R. (2004). Cooccurring alcohol and cocaine dependence: recent findings from clinical and field studies. *Alcohol Clin. Exp. Res.* 28, 976–981.

Fingarette H. (1988) Heavy Drinking: The Myth of Alcoholism as a Disease. Berkeley, CA: University of California Press.

Finn PR, Sharkansky EJ, Brandt KM, Turcotte N. (2000). The effects of familial risk, personality, and expectancies on alcohol use and abuse. *Journal of Abnormal Psychology.* 109:122–133.

Finney JW, Monahan SC. (1996) The cost effectiveness of treatment for alcoholism: A second approximation. *Journal of Studies on Alcohol;* 57: 229-243.

Fishbein DH; Krupitsky E; Flannery BA; Langevin DJ; Bobashev G; Verbitskaya E; Augustine CB; Bolla KI; Zvartau E; Schech B; Egorova V; Bushara N; Tsoy M. (2007) Neurocognitive characterizations of Russian heroin addicts without a significant history of other drug use. *Drug Alcohol Depend;* 90(1):25-38.

Grant I, Judd LL (1976) Neuropsychological and EEG disturbances in polydrug users. *Am. J. Psychiatry.* Sep; 133(9):1039-42.

Gelb, A. M., Richman, B. L., & Anand, O. P. (1978). Quantitative and temporal relationships of alcohol use in narcotic addicts and methadone maintenance patients undergoing alcohol detoxification. *American Journal of Drug and Alcohol Abuse.* 5, 191–198.

Gitto S., Micco L., Conti F., Andreone P. and Bernardi M. Alcohol and viral hepatitis: A mini-review : *Dig. Liver Dis.* 2009 Jan;41(1):67-70.

Goeders NE. (2003) The impact of stress on addiction. *European Neuropsychopharmacology,* 13: 435–441.

Gonzalez R, Rippeth JD, Carey CL et al. (2004) Neurocognitive performance of methamphetamine users discordant for history of marijuana exposure. *Drug Alcohol Depend;* 76:181:190.

Goodwin, D.W.; Schulsinger, F.; Hermansen, L.; Guze, S.B.; & Winokur, G. (1973) Alcohol problems in adoptees raised apart from alcoholic biological parents. *Archives of General Psychiatry.* 28:238-243.

Goodwin D.W.; Crane J.B, Guze S.B. (1969) Phenomenological aspects of the alcoholic "blackout." *British Journal of Psychiatry;* 115:1033-1038.

Gossop, M. (1996). Cognitive and behavioural treatments for substance misuse. In Edwards G. & Dare C. (Ed.), *Psychotherapy, Psychological Treatments and the Addictions* (158-172). Great Britain. Cambridge University Press.

Gossop, M., Marsden, J., Stewart, D. et al. (1998), 'Substance use, health and social problems of clients at 54 drug treatment agencies: intake data from the National Treatment Outcome Research Study (NTORS)', *British Journal of Psychiatry.* 173, pp. 166–71.

Gossop, M., Marsden, J., Stewart, D., & Rolfe, A. (2000). Patterns of improvement after methadone treatment: 1 year follow-up results from the National Treatment Outcome Research Study. *Drug and Alcohol Dependence.* 60, 275–286.

Gossop, M. (2001). A web of dependence. *Addiction.* 96, 677–678.

Gossop M, Marsden J, Stewart D. (2002a) Dual dependence: assessment of dependence upon alcohol and illicit drugs, and the relationship of alcohol dependence among drug misusers to patterns of drinking, illicit drug use and health problems. *Addiction.* 97:169–78.

Gossop, M., Marsden, J., Stewart, D., Kidd, T. (2002b). Changes in use of crack cocaine after drug misuse treatment: 4–5 year follow-up results from the National Treatment Outcome Research Study NTORS. *Drug Alcohol Depend.* 66, 21–28.

Gossop, M., Stewart, D., Browne, N., & Marsden, J. (2003). Methadone treatment for opiate dependent patients in general practice and specialist clinic settings: Outcomes at 2-year follow-up. *Journal of Substance Abuse Treatment.* 24, 313– 321.

Gossop M, Marsden J, Stewart D, Kidd T. (2003) The National Treatment Outcome Research Study (NTORS): 4–5 year follow-up results. *Addiction*; 98: 291–303.

Gossop M, Stewart D, Marsden J. (2006) Effectiveness of drug and alcohol counselling during methadone treatment: content, frequency, and duration of counselling and association with substance use outcomes. *Addiction.* 101, 404–12.

Granfield R, Cloud W. (1999) Coming clean: Overcoming addiction without treatment. New York: New York University Press.

Green, J., & Jaffe, J. H. (1977). Alcohol and opiate dependence; a review. *Journal of Studies on Alcohol.* 38, 1274– 1293.

Guerra D, Sole A, Cami J, Tobena A. (1987) Neuropsychological performance in opiate addicts after rapid detoxification. *Drug Alcohol Depend;* 20:261:270.

Haaga DAF, McCrady B, Lebow J. (2006) Integrative Principles for Treating Substance Use Disorders. *Journal of Clinical Psychology;* 62 (6): 675–684.

Harper C, Matsumoto I. Ethanol and brain damage. *Current opinion in Pharmacology.* 2005; 5:73-78.

Hartel, D. M., Schoenbaum, E. E., Selwyn, P. A., Kline, J., Davenny, K., Klein, R. S., et al. (1995). Heroin use during methadone maintenance treatment: The importance of methadone dose and cocaine use. *American Journal of Public Health.* 85, 83– 88.

Hartzler B, Fromme K. (2003) Fragmentary blackouts: Their etiology and effect on alcohol expectancies. *Alcoholism: Clinical and Experimental Research.* Vol.27, No.4: 628-637.

Hester R, Garavan H (2004) Executive dysfunction in cocaine addiction: evidence for discordant frontal, cingulate, and cerebellar activity. *J. Neurosci.* 24:11017–11022

Hester R. K. & Miller W.R. (2003). *Handbook of Alcoholism Treatment Approaches.* USA. Pearson Education Inc..

Hillebrand, J., Marsden, J., Finch, E., & Strang, J. (2001). Excessive alcohol consumption and drinking expectations among clients in methadone maintenance. *Journal of Substance Abuse Treatment.* 21, 155–160.

Hillemacher T, Bayerlein K, Wilhelm J, Bönsch D, Poleo D, Sperling W, Kornhuber J, Bleich S. (2006) Recurrent detoxifications are associated with craving in patients classified as type I according to Lesch's typology. *Alcohol and Alcoholism.* 41(1), 66-69.

Hillemacher, T. and Bleich, S. (2008) Neurobiology and treatment in alcoholism--recent findings regarding Lesch's typology of alcohol dependence. *Alcohol and Alcoholism.* 43, 341-6.

Hodge DR, Cardenas P, Montoya H. (2001) Substance use: spirituality and religious participation as protective factors among rural youths. *Social Work Research,* 25(3): 153–160.

Hser, Y. I., Anglin, M. D., & Powers, K. (1990). Longitudinal patterns of alcohol use by narcotics addicts. *Recent Developments in Alcoholism*. 8,145– 171.

Hser YI, Hoffman V, Grella CE, Anglin MD. (2001) A 33-year follow-up of narcotics addicts. *Arch. Gen. Psychiatry*. 58, 503 – 8.

Hubbard, R., Craddock, S., Flynn, P., Anderson, J., Etheridge, R., (1997). Overview of 1 year follow-up outcomes in the Drug Abuse Treatment Outcome Study DATOS. *Psychol. Addict. Behav.* 11, 261–278.

Hunt, D.E., Strug, D.L., Goldsmith, D.S., Lipton, D.S., Robertson, K., & Truitt, L. (1986). Alcohol use and abuse: Heavy drinking among methadone clients. *American Journal of Drug and Alcohol Abuse*. 12, 147–164.

Ives, R. and Ghelani, P. (2006), 'Polydrug use (the use of drugs in combination): a brief review', *Drugs: Education, Prevention and Policy,* 13, pp. 225–32.

Jellinek EM. Phases in the drinking history of alcholics: analysis of a survey conducted by the official organ of Alcoholics Anonymous. *Q. J. Stud. Alcohol.* 1946; (7), 1-88.

Jiang ZN, Wang WP. (1992) Drug abuse. Beijing: *Technology Publishing Company,* 119-209.

John, D., Kwiatkowski, C., Booth, R. (2001). Differences among out-of-treatment drug injectors who use stimulants only, opiates only or both: implications for treatment entry. *Drug Alcohol Depend.* 64, 165–172.

Johnson BA, Ait-Daoud N. (2000) Neuropharmacological treatments for alcoholism: scientific basis and clinical findings. *Psychopharmacology*. 149, 327–44.

Jones, B. T. and McMahon, J. (1992) Negative and positive expectancies in lone and group problem drinkers. *British Journal of Addiction*. 87, 929–930.

Joseph H, Appel P. (1985) Alcoholism and methadone treatment: consequences for the patient and program. *Am. J. Drug Alcohol Abuse*. 11:37–53.

Kabat-Zinn, J. (1982) An outpatient program in behavioral medicine for chronic pain patients based on the practice of mindfulness meditation: Theoretical considerations and preliminary results. *General Hospital Psychiatry;* 4: 33–47.

Kabat-Zinn J, Chapman A, Salmon P. (1997) The relationship of cognitive and somatic components of anxiety to patient preference for alternative relaxation techniques. *Mind/Body Medicine;* 2: 101–109.

Kaplan MS, Marks G, et al. (1997) Distress and coping among women with HIV infection: Preliminary findings from a multiethnic sample. *American Journal of Orthopsychiatry;* 67(1): 80–91.

Kaufman, E. (1982). The relationship of alcoholism and alcohol abuse to the abuse of other drugs. *American Journal of Drug and Alcohol Abuse*. 9, 1–17.

Kelly GA. (1955) The Psychology of Personal Constructs. New York: Norton.

Kendler KS, Gardner CO, et al. (1997) Religion, psychopathology, and substance use and abuse: A multimeasure, genetic-epidemiologic study. *American Journal of Psychiatry;* 154(3): 322–329.

Khantzian EJ. (1980) An ego-self theory of substance dependence. In Lettieri DJ, Sayers M. & Wallensterin HW (eds), Theories of addiction. NIDA Research Monograph No. 30 DHHS Publication No. ADM 80-967. Washington DC: Superintendent of Documents, U.S. Government Printing Office, 1980.

Khantzian EJ. (1985) The self-medication hypothesis of addictive disorders: Focus on heroin and cocaine dependence. Am J Psychiatry;142: 1259-64.

Khantzian EJ, Halliday KS, McAuliffe WE. (1990) Addiction and the vulnerable self. New York: Guilford Press.

Kokavec A, Crowe S.(1999) A comparison of cognitive performance in binge versus regular chronic alcohol misusers. *Alcohol and Alcoholism;* Vol.24, pp.601-608.

Kosten TR, Rounsaville BJ, Kleber HD. (1986) A 2.5 year follow-up of depressions, life crises, and treatment effects on abstinence among opioid addicts. *Archives of General Psychiatry,* 43: 733–739.

Kreek MJ. (1978) Medical complications between opiates and alcohol. *Ann. N.Y. Acad. Sci.* 362, 36 – 49.

Kreek, M. J. (1984). Opioid interactions with alcohol. *Advances in Alcohol & Substance Abuse.* 3, 35–46.

Kreek, M.J. (1990). Drug interactions in humans related to drug abuse and its treatment. *Modern Methods in Pharmacology.* 6, 265–282.

Krupitsky E, Burakov A, Romanova T, Dunaevsky I, Strassman R, Grinenko A. (2002) Ketamine psychotherapy for heroin addiction: immediate effects and two-year follow-up. *Journal of Substance Abuse Treatment;* 23: 273– 283.

Laudet AB, Morgen K, White WL. (2006) The role of social supports, spirituality, religiousness, life meaning and affiliation with 12-step fellowships in quality of life satisfaction among individuals in recovery from alcohol and drug problems. *Alcohol Treatment Quarterly;* 24(1–2): 33–73.

Leri, F., Bruneau, J., Stewart, J. (2003). Understanding polydrug use: review of heroin and cocaine co-use. *Addiction.* 98, 7–22.

Lesch, O. M., Dietzel, M., Musalek, M., Walter, H. and Zeiler, K (1988). The course of alcoholism. Long-term prognosis in different Types. *Forensic Science International.* 36, 121–138.

Lesch O, Riegler A, Gutierrez K, Hertling I, Ramskogler K, Semler B, Zoghlami A, Benda N, Walter H (2001). The European Acamprosate Trials: conclusions for research and therapy. *J. Biomed. Sci.* 8, 89-95.

Liang JH, Ren YH. (2001) The study on drug abuse's addicted mechanism, epidemiology, prevention and cure. *Chinese Journal of Drug Depend;* 10(1): 2-8.

Litt MD, Babor TF, DelBoca FK, Kadden RM and Cooney NL (1992) Types of alcoholics: II. Application of an empirically derived typology of treatment matching, *Archives of General Psychiatry.* **49**, 609–614.

Litt, M.D., Cooney, N.L. & Morse, P. (2000). Reactivity to alcohol-related stimuli in the laboratory and in the field: predictors of craving in treated alcoholics. *Addiction.* 95, 889-900.

Lotfi J, Meyer JS.(1989) Cerebral hemodynamic and metabolic effects of chronic alcoholism. *Cerebrovasc Brain Metabolism Rev;* 1:2-25.

Lowman, R., Allen, J., Stout, R. L., & Relapse Research Group (1996). Marlatt's taxonomy of relapse precipitants: Overview of procedures and results. *Addiction.* 91, 51–72.

Lyoo IK, Pollack MH, Silveri MM et al. (2006) Prefrontal and temporal gray matter density decreases in opiate dependence. *Psychopharmacology;* 184:139:144.

Lykouras L, Moussas G, Botsis (2004) Examination of type I/II alcoholism typology in a Greek hospital treatment population. *European Psychiatry* 19, 214-218.

Maddux, J. F., & Elliot, B. (1975). Problem drinkers among patients on methadone. *American Journal of Alcohol Abuse.* 2, 245– 254.

Magura, S., Nwakeze, P.C.& Demsky S.Y. (1998). Preditors of Treatment Retention in Methadone Treatment. *Addiction.* 93, 51-60.

Malcolm, B., Hesselbrock, M., Segal, B. (2006). Multiple substance dependence and course of alcoholism among Alaska native men and women. *Subst. Use Misuse.* 51, 729–741.

Mann K, Agartz I, Shoaf S, Momenam R, Hommer DW, Sullivan EV, Drobes DJ, George MK, Bares R, Mundle G, Heinz A (2001). Neuroimaging in alcoholism: ethanol and brain damage. *Alcoholism: Clinical and Experimental Research;* Vol. 25, No5, pp 104-109.

Maremmani, I., Pani, P.P., Mellini, A., Pacini, M., Marini, G., Lovrecic, M., Perugi, G., Shinderman, M., (2007). Alcohol and cocaine use and abuse among opioid addicts engaged in a methadone maintenance treatment program. *J. Addict. Dis.* 26 (1), 61–70.

Margolin A, Beitel M, Schuman-Olivier Z, Avants SK. (2006) A controlled study of a spirituality-focused intervention for increasing motivation for HIV prevention among drug users. *AIDS Education & Prevention;* 18(4): 311–322.

Marlatt, G. A. & Gordon, J. R. (Eds.) (1985). Relapse prevention: Maintenance strategies in the treatment of addiction behaviour. New York: Guilford Press

Marlatt, G. A. & Roseenow, D. J. (1980) Cognitive processses in alcohol use: expectancy and the alanced placebo design, in: N. K. Mello (Ed.) *Advances in Substance Abuse: behavioral and biological research.* 1, 159-199 (Greenwich, CT, JAI Press)

Marlatt GA, Witkiewitz K, Dillworth TM, Bowen SW, Parks GA, Macpherson LM. (2004) Vipassana meditation as a treatment for alcohol and drug use disorders. In S. C. Hayes, V. M. Follette, & M. M. Linehanm (Eds.), *Mindfulness and acceptance: Expanding the cognitive-behavioral tradition* (pp. 261–287). New York: Guilford Press.

Marsden J, Eastwood B, Bradbury C, Dale-Perera A, Farrell M, et al. (2009) Effectiveness of community treatments for heroin and crack cocaine addiction in England: a prospective, in-treatment cohort study. *Lancet;* 374: 1262–70.

Martin, C. S., Clifford, P. R., Maisto, S. A. Earleywine M, Kirlsci L, Longabaugh R. (1996) Polydrug use in an inpatient treatment sample of problem drinkers. *Alcoholism: Clinical and Experimental Research.* 20, 413–417.

Mattick, R. P., Breen, C., Kimber, J., & Davoli, M. (2003). Methadone maintenance therapy versus no opioid replacement therapy for opioid dependence. *Cochrane Database of Systematic,* 2.

Maxwell, S., & Shinderman, M. (1999). Optimizing response to methadone maintenance treatment: Use of higher-dose methadone. *Journal of Psychoactive Drugs*. 31, 95– 102.

Medina, K., Shear, P. (2007). Anxiety, depression, and behavioural symptoms of executive dysfunction in ecstasy users: contributions of polydrug use. *Drug Alcohol Depend.* 87, 303–311.

Melgaard B, Henriksen L, Ahlgren P, Danielsen UT, Sorensen H, Paulson OB. (1993) Regional cerebral blood flow in chronic alcoholics measured by single photon emission on computerized tomography. *Acta Neurologica Scandinavica;* 82, 87-93.

McLellan, A.T., Luborsky, L., O'Brien, C.P. & Woody, G.E. (1980). An improved diagnostic instrument for substance abuse patients: The Addiction Severity Index. *Journal of Nervous & Mental Diseases,* 168, 26-33.

McLellan AT, Grissom GR, Zanis D, Randall M, Brill P, O'Brien CP. (1997) Problemservice 'matching' in addiction treatment. A prospective study in 4 programs. *Archives of General Psychiatry;* 54: 730–735.

Miller WR, Zweben A, DiClemente CC, Rychtarik RG. (1992) Motivational enhancement therapy manual: a clinical research guide for therapists treating individuals with alcohol abuse and dependence (Vol. 2, Project MATCH Monograph Series). Rockville, MD: National Institute on Alcohol Abuse and Alcoholism.

Miller, W.R., Tonigan, J.S. & Longabaugh, R. (1995). The Drinker Inventory of Consequences (DrInC): An Instrument for Assessing Adverse Consequences of Alcohol Abuse. Project MATCH Monograph Series, Vol. 4. DHHS Publication No. 95-3911. Rockville, MD: National Institute on Alcohol Abuse and Alcoholism.

Miller JJ, Fletcher K, Kabat-Zinn J. (1995) Three-year follow-up and clinical implications of a mindfulness meditation-based stress reduction intervention in the treatment of anxiety disorders. *General Hospital Psychiatry;* 17: 192–200.

Miller, W. R., & Tonigan, J. S. (1996). Assessing drinkers' motivation for change: The Stages of Change Readiness and Treatment Eagerness Scale (SOCRATES). *Psychology of Addictive Behaviors,* 10, 81–89.

Miller WR, Brown SA. (1997) Why psychologists should treat alcohol and drug problems. *American Psychologist;* 52: 1269-1279.

Miller WR. (1998) Researching the spiritual dimensions of alcohol and other drug problems. Addiction; 93: 979–990.

Miller L, Davies M, Greenwald S. (2000) Religiosity and substance use and abuse among adolescents in the national comorbidity survey. *Journal of the American Academy of Child and Adolescent Psychiatry;* 39(9): 1190–1197.

Modell, J.G., Glaser, F.B., Mountz, J.M., Schmaltz S. & Cyr, L. (1992). Obsessive and compulsive characteristics of alcohol abuse and dependence: Quantification by a newly developed questionnaire. *Alcoholism: Clinical Experimental Research,* 16, 266-271.

Molina JA, Bermejo F, del Ser T, Jimenez-Jimenez FJ, Herranz A, Fernandez-Calle P, Ortuno B, Sainz MJ. (1994) Alcoholic cognitive deterioration and nutritional deficiencies. *Acta Neurologia Scandinavica;* 89, 384-390.

Moos RH. (2003) Addictive disorders in context: Principles and puzzles of effective treatment and recovery. *Psychology of Addictive Behaviors;* 17: 3–12.

Moos, R (2005). Iatrogenic effects of psychosocial interventions for substance use disorders: prevalence, predictors, prevention. *Addiction.* **100, 595 – 604.**

Morel A, Hervé F, Fontaine B. (1998) Abordagens Psicológicas. In Morel A, Hervé F, Fontaine B (eds) *Cuidados ao toxicodependente.* Lisboa: Climepsi Editores.

Morgenstern J, Leeds J. (1993) Contemporary psychoanalytic theories of substance abuse: A disorder in search of a paradigm. *Psychotherapy;* 30: 194-206.

National Treatment Agency for Substance Misuse. (2006) Models of care for adult drug misusers: update. http://www.nta.nhs.uk/ publications/ documents/nta_modelsofcare_update_2006_moc3.pdf

National Institute on Alcohol Abuse and Alcoholism (1995). The Physician's Guide to Helping Patients with Alcohol Problems. US DHHS NIH Publ. No. 95-3769. Washington, DC: PHS.

Nava F, Manzato E, Leonardi C, Lucchini A. (2008) Opioid maintenance therapy suppresses alcohol intake in heroin addicts with alcohol dependence: Preliminary results of an open randomized study. *Progress in Neuro-Psychopharmacology & Biological Psychiatry* 32, 1867–1872.

Neff JA, Shorkey CT, Windsor LC. (2006) Contrasting faith-based and traditional substance abuse treatment programs. *Journal of Substance Abuse Treatment;* 30: 49–61.

Nelson EC, Heath AC, Bucholz KK, Madden PA, Fu Q, Knopik V, Lynskey MT, Whitfield JB, Statham DJ, Martin NG (2004). Genetic epidemiology of alcohol-induced blackouts. *Archives of General Psychiatry.* Vol.61, pp. 257-263.

Oei TPS, Baldwin AR (1994) Expectancy theory: A two-process model of alcohol use and abuse. *Journal of Studies on Alcohol.* 55, 525-534.

Oei TPS, Fergusson S, Lee NK. (1998) The differential role of alcohol expectancies and drinking refusal self efficacy in problem and nonproblem drinkers. *Journal of Studies on Alcohol.* 59, 704–11.

O'Grady, K., Arria, A., Fitzelle, D. & Wish, E. (2008), 'Heavy Drinking and Polydrug Use among College Students', *Journal of Drug Issues*, 38(2), pp. 445-466.

O'Mahony, J. (2004) A Comparison of Alcohol Abusers who have and have not Experienced Blackouts. *European Addiction Research;* 10(3): pp. 95-98.

O'Leary MR, Donovan DM, Chaney EF. (1979) Cognitive impairment and treatment outcome in alcoholics: preliminary findings. *Journal of Clinical Psychiatry;* 40, 397-398.

Olievenstein C. (1982) A Vida do Toxicómano. Rio de Janeiro: Zahar.

Olivenstein C. (1987) La Dependence: Un Phénomène Psychique Actif in Olivenstrein C, Angel P, Géraud B, Mège JY, Perpére A, Petit P, Valleur M. La Clinique du Toxicomane, Paris, Editions Universitaires, p. 13-24.

Oorsouw KV, Merckelbach H, Ravelli D, Nijman H, Mekking-Pompen I.(2004) Alcoholic blackout for criminally relevant behavior. *The Journal of the American Academy of Psychiatry and the Law;* 32, pp. 364-70.

Ornstein TJ, Iddon JL, Baldacchino AM et al. (2000) Profiles of cognitive dysfunction in chronic amphetamine and heroin abusers. *Neuropsychopharmacology;* 23:113:126.

Oscar-Berman M, Kirkley SM, Gansler DA, Couture A.(2004) Comparisons of Korsakoff and non-Korsakoff alcoholics on neuropsychological tests of prefrontal brain functioning. *Alcohol: Clinical and Experimental Research;* 28(4):667-75.

Ottomanelli, G. (1992). *HIV infectionand intravenous drug use.* Westport, CT: Praeger

Ottomanelli G. (1999) Methadone patients and alcoho abuse. *J. Subst. Abuse Treat.* 16, 113–21.

Pagès-Berthier J. (2002) Personalidade e toxicomania: abordagem psicanalítica. *In* Angel P, Richard D, & Valleur M. (Eds.). *Toxicomanias* (pp. 179-185). Lisboa: Climepsi Editores.

Pandey, G.N., Fawcett, J., Gibbons, R., Clark, D.C., David, J.M. (1988) Platelet monoamine oxidase in alcoholism. *Biological Psychiatry.* 24, 15-24.

Pardini DA, Plante TG, et al. (2000) Religious faith and spirituality in substance abuse recovery: Determining the mental health benefits. *Journal of Substance Abuse Treatment;* 19(4): 347–354.

Patterson, T., Semple, S., Zians, J., Strathdee, S. (2005). Methamphetamineusing HIV-positive men who have sex with men: correlates of polydrug use. *J. Urban Health.* 82 (Suppl. 1), 120–126.

Pau CW, Lee TM, Chan SF. (2002) The impact of heroin on frontal executive functions. *Arch. Clin. Neuropsychol;* 17:663: 670.

Pessione F, Gerchstein JL, Rueff B. (1995) Parental history of alcoholism: a risk factor for alcohol related peripheral neuropathies. *Alcohol and Alcoholism;* 30, 749-754.

Pinto Gouveia, J., Ramalheira, C., Robalo, M., Borges, J. Almeida; J. (1993). Inventário de expectativas e crenças pessoais acerca do álcool. Psiquiatria Clínica 14, 147-163.

Pombo, S., Reizinho, R., Ismail, F., Barbosa, A., Luísa Figueira, M., Neves Cardoso, J.M., Lesch, O.M. (2007). NETER Alcoholic 5 Subtypes: Validity with Lesch 4 Evolutionary Subtypes. *International Journal of Psychiatry in Clinical Practice,* 1-10.

Poikolainen K.(1982) Blackouts increase with age, social class and the frequency of intoxication. *Acta Neurol. Scand;* 66, 555-560.

Pombo, S., Reizinho, R., Ismail, F. & Neves Cardoso. J,M, (2008a). Denegação do alcoolismo nos subtipos I e II de Cloninger. *Análise Psicológica,* XXVI, 59-69.

Pombo, S., Levy, P., Bicho, M., Ismail, F., Cardoso, J.M.(2008b) Neuropsychological function and platelet monoamine oxidase activity levels in type I alcoholic patients. *Alcohol Alcohol.* 43, 423–30.

Pombo S, Lesch OM. (2009) The alcoholic phenotypes among different multidimensional typologies: similarities and their classification procedures. *Alcohol Alcohol.* 44, 46-54

Pombo, S., Ismail, F. & Neves Cardoso. J,M. "Cravers" pelo álcool. *Revista Psicologia, Saúde & Doenças* (in press)

Pope HG Jr, Gruber AJ, Hudson JI, Cohane G, Huestis MA, Yurgelun-Todd D.(2003) Early-onset cannabis use and cognitive deficits: what is the nature of the association? Dr*ug* Alcohol Depend; 69:303:310.

Prescott, C.A., and Kendler, K.S (1999). Genetic and environmental contributions to alcohol abuse and dependence in a population–based sample of male twins. American Journal of Psychiatry. 156: 34–40.

Prochaska, J.O. & DiClemente, C.C. (1986). Toward a comprehensive model of change. In W. Miller and N. Heather (Eds.), Addictive behaviours: Processes of Change. New York: Plenum Press, 3-28.

Rado S. (1933) The psychoanalysis of pharmacotymias. *Psychoanal Q*; 2:1-23.

Rask MB, Jørgensen T, Jensen JP, Jørgensen KB, Madsen M, Nielsen B, et al. (2006) Influence of Pretreatment Coping Strategies on the Outcome of Outpatient Treatment of Danish Alcohol Abusers. *European Addiction Research;* 12: 83–90.

Ratti MT, Soragna D, Sibilla L, Giardini A, Albergati A, Savoldi F, Bo P. (1999) Cognitive impairment and cerebral atrophy in "heavy drinkers". *Neuro-psychopharmacology and biology psychiatry;* vol.23, pp- 243-258.

Rodríguez M.(1993) Cognitive functioning in male polydrug abusers with and without family history of alcoholism. *Percept Mot. Skills.* Oct;77(2):483-8.

Roehrich L and Goldman MS. (1993) Experience-dependent neuropsychological recovery and the treatment of alcoholism. *J. Cons. Clin. Psychology;* (5), 812-21.

Room R, Babor T, Rehm J (2005). Alcohol and public health. *Lancet,* 365:519–529

Rosa A. (1994) Toxicodependência: as desintoxicações ultra-rápidas. Coimbra: [s.n], 94(2).

Rourke SB, Loberg T. (1996) Neurobiological correlates of alcoholism. In Grant I, Adams KM. Neuropsychological assessment of neuropsychiatric disorders; New York, USM, Oxford University Press.

Rollnick, S., Heather, N., Gold, R. and Hall, W. (1992) Development of a short 'readiness to change' questionnaire for use in brief, opportunistic interventions among excessive drinkers. *British Journal of Addiction* 87, 743–754.

Roszell, D. K., Calsyn, D. A., & Chaney, E. F. (1986). Alcohol use and psychopathology in opioid addicts on methadone maintenance. *American Journal of Drug and Alcohol Abuse* 12, 269– 278.

Rounsaville, B.J., Weissman, M.M., & Kleber, H.D. (1982). The significance of alcoholism in treated opiate addicts. *Journal of Nervous and Mental Disease* 170, 479–488.

Rowan-Szal, G. A., Chatham, L. R., & Simpson, D. D. (2000). Importance of identifying cocaine and alcohol dependent methadone clients. *American Journal on Addictions* 9, 38–50.

Rinn W, Desai N, Rosenblatt H, Gastfriend DR (2002). Addiction denial and cognitive dysfunction: a preliminary investigation. *J. Neuropsychiatry Clin Neuroscience.* 14, 52-57.

Rittmannsberger H, Silberbauer C, Lehner R, Ruschak M. (2000) Alcohol consumption during methadone maintenance treatment. *Eur. Addict. Res.* 6:2–7.

Ryback RS.(1970) Alcohol amnesia: observations in seven drinking inpatient alcoholics. *Q. J. Stud. Alcohol;* 31, 616-632.

Rubonis, A.V., Colby, S.M., Monti, P.M., Rosenow, D.J., Gulliver, S.B. & Sirota, A.D. (1994). Alcohol cue reactivity and mood induction in male and female alcoholics. *Journal Studies Alcohol.* 55, 487-494.

Saitz, Richard (2007). Treatment of Alcohol and Other Drug Dependence. *Liver Transplantation.* 13, 59-64.

Schiff, E. R. (1997). Hepatitis C and alcohol. *Hepatology.* 26, 39S– 42S.

Schottenfeld, R. S., Pakes, J. R., & Kosten, T. R. (1998). Prognostic factors in buprenorphine-versus methadone-maintained patients. *Journal of Nervous and Mental Disease.* 186, 35–43.

Schut, J., File, K., & Wohlmuth, T. (1973). Alcohol use by narcotic addicts in methadone maintenance treatment. *Quarterly Journal of Studies on Alcohol.* 34, 1356– 1359.

Selzer M.L. (1971). The Michigan Alcoholism Screening Test (MAST): the quest for a new diagnostic instrument. *American Journal Psychiatry.* 127, 1653– 1658.

Senbanjo R, Wolff K, Marshall J. (2006) Excessive alcohol consumption is associated with reduced quality of life among methadone patients. *Addiction;* 102:257–63.

Serra A.V., Lima M.M. (1979). O uso do «Michigan Alcoholism Screening Test» como instrumento discriminador entre grupos de alcoólicos e de não-alcoólicos. *Coimbra Médica.* 197, 39-5.

Silvers JM, Tokunaga S, Berry RB, White AM, Mattews DB. (2003) Impairments in spatial learning and memory: ethanol, allopregnanolone, and the hippocampus. *Brain Research Reviews;* 43, 275-284.

Simpson D., George J. & Grace A. (1997). Drug Abuse Treatment Retention and Process Effects on Follow-up Outcomes. *Drug and Alcohol Dependence,* 47, 227-235.

Sinha R, Fuse T, Aubin LR, O'Malley SS. (2000) Psychological stress, drug-related cues, and cocaine craving. *Psychopharmacology;* 152: 140–148.

Sklar S. M; Annis H. M.; Turner N. E. (1997) Development and validation of the Drug-Taking Confidence Questionnaire: A measure of coping self-efficacy. *Addictive behaviors.* 22, 655-670.

Skinner H (1982) The Drug Abuse Screening Test. *Addictive Behaviors.* 7:363–371

Sobell, L. C., & Sobell, M. B. (2003). Alcohol consumption measures. In J. P. Allen & V. Wilson (Eds.), *Assessing alcohol problems* (2nd ed.) (pp. 75-99). Rockville, MD: National Institute on Alcohol Abuse and Alcoholism.

Solowij N, Stephens RS, Roffman RA et al. (2002) Cognitive functioning of long-term heavy cannabis users seeking treatment. *JAMA;* 287:1123:1131.

Soyka M, Zingg C, Koller G, Kuefner H. (2008) Retention rate and substance use in methadone and buprenorphine maintenance therapy and predictors of outcome: results. *Int. J. Neuropsychopharmacol.* 21, 1-13.

Southwick, L., Steele, C., Marlatt, G. A., & Lindell, M. (1981). Alcohol-related expectancies: Defined by phase of intoxication and drinking experience. *Journal of Consulting and Clinical Psychology,* 49, 713-721.

Srivastava, A., Kahan, M., Ross, S. (2008). The effect of methadone maintenance treatment on alcohol consumption: a systematic review. *J. Subst. Abuse Treat.* 34, 215–223.

Stacy AW, Widaman KF, Marlatt GA. (1990) Expectancy models of alcohol use. *Journal of Personality and Social Psychology.* 58:918–928.

Staines, G. L., Magura, S., Foote, J. et al. (2001) Polysubstance use among alcoholics. *Journal of Addictive Diseases.* 20, 53–69.

Stevens A, Peschk I, Schwarz J. (2007) Implicit learning, executive function and hedonic activity in chronic polydrug abusers, currently abstinent polydrug abusers and controls. *Addiction.* Jun;102(6):937-46.

Strang, J., Griffiths, P., & Powis, B. (1999). Fountain, J., Williamson, S., & Gossop, M. (1999) Which drugs cause overdose among opiate misusers? Study of personal and witnessed overdoses. *Drug and Alcohol Review.* 18, 253– 261.

Strang, J., Marsden, J., Cummins, M., Farrell, M., Finch, E., Gossop, M., Stewart D, Welch S. (2000). Randomized trial of supervised injectable versus oral methadone maintenance: Report of feasibility and 6-month outcome. *Addiction.* 95, 1631– 1645.

Stein MD, Cioe P, Friedmann PD. (2005) Buprenorphine retention in primary care. *J. Gen. Intern. Med.* 20(11), 1038-41.

Stenbacka, M., Beck, O., Leifman, A., Romelsjo, A., Helander, A. (2007). Problem drinking in relation to treatment outcome among opiate addicts in methadone maintenance treatment. *Drug Alcohol Rev.* 26, 55–63.

Stimmel, B., Vernace, S., & Tobias, H. (1972). Hepatic dysfunction in heroin addicts. The role of alcohol. *Journal of the American Medical Association.* 222, 811 – 812.

Sullivan, J.L., Baenziger, J.C., Wagner, D.L. (1990) Platelet MAO in subtypes of alcoholism. *Biological Psychiatry.* 27, 911-922.

Sullivan EV, Rosenbloom MJ, Pfefferbaum A. (2000) Pattern of cognitive and motor deficits in detoxified alcoholic men. *Alcoholism: Clinical and Experimental Research.* 2000, 24:611-621.

Sullivan EV, Fama R, Pferfferbaum M. (2002) A profile of neuropsychological deficits in alcoholic women. *Neuropsychology;* Vol.16, No.1, pp. 74-83.

Sumnall, H., Wagstaff, G., Cole, J. (2004). Self-reported psychopathology in polydrug users. J. *Psychopharmacol.* 18, 75–82.

Tarter, RE, Schneider DU. (1976) Blackouts: Relationship with memory capacity and alcoholism history. *Arch. Gen. Psychiatry;* 33:1492-1496.

Taylor PJ, Kopelman MD.(1984) Amnesia for criminal offenses. *Psychol. Med;* 14, 581-8.

Teplin, D., Raz, B., Daiter, J., Varenbut, M., Plater-Zyberk, C. (2007). Screening for alcohol use patterns among methadone maintenance patients. *Am. J. Drug Alcohol Abuse.* 33, 179–183.

Toates F. (1998) The interaction of cognitive and stimulus – response processes in the control of behaviour. *Neurosci. Biobehav. Rev*; 22: 59–83.

Turner, N. E., Annis, H. M., & Sklar, S. M. (1997). Measurement of Antecedents to Drug and Alcohol Use: Psychometric Properties of the Inventory of Drug-Taking Situations (IDTS). *Behav. Res. Ther.* 35, N. 5.

Verkes RJ, Gijsman HJ, Pieters MSM, Schoemaker RC, de Visser S, Kuijpers M, Pennings EJM, de Bruin D, Van de Wijngaart G, Van Gerven JMA, Cohen AF (2001) Cognitive performance and serotonergic function in users of ecstasy. *Psychopharmacology.* 153:196–202.

Volkow ND, Fowler JS, Wang GJ (1999) Imaging studies on the role of dopamine in cocaine reinforcement and addiction in humans. J. *Psychopharmacol.* 13:337–345

von Knorring, A. L., Bohman, M., von Knorring, L. and Oreland, L. (1985) Platelet MAO activity as a biological marker in subgroups of alcoholism. *Acta Psychiatrica Scandinavica.* 72, 51–58.

von Knorring, A.L., Hallman, J., von Knorring, L., Oreland, L. (1998) Platelet monoamine oxidase activity in type 1 and type 2 alcoholism. *Alcoholism: Clinical and Experimental Research.* 22, 598-604.

Waldrop A, Back S, Verduin M, Brady K. (2007).Triggers for cocaine and alcohol use in the presence and absence of posttraumatic. *Addictive behaviors.* 32, 634-9.

Walter H; Ramskogler-Skala K; Dvorak A; Gutierrez-Lobos K; Hartl D; Hertling I; Munda P; Thau K; Lesch O; Witte P (2006) Glutamic acidin withdrawal and weaning in patients classified according to Cloninger´s and Lesch´s typologies. *Alcohol & Alcoholism* 41, 505-511.

Waltman D. (1995) Key Ingredients to Effective Addictions Treatment. *Journal of Substance Abuse Treatment;* 12 (6): 429-439.

Weaver GD, Turner NH, O'Dell KJ. (2000) Depressive symptoms, stress, and coping among women recovering from addiction. *Journal of Substance Abuse Treatment;* 18: 161–167.

West, S L, O'Neal, K K, Graham, C W. (2000) A meta-analysis comparing the effectiveness of buprenorphine and methadone. *J-Subst-Abuse.* 12(4), 405-14.

Westreich LM. (2005) Alcohol and mental illness: clinical focus. *Prim. Psychiatry.* 12:41–6.

World Health Organization (2004).Global status report: alcohol policy. Geneva.

World Health Organization, WHO (1994). International Statistical Classification of Diseases and Related Health Problems. Tenth Revision. Geneva: WHO.

White AM, Simson PE, Best PJ.(1997) Comparison between the effects of ethanol and diazepam on spatial working memory in the rat. *Psychopharmacology;* 133:256-261.

White AM, Jamieson-Drake D, Swartzwelder HS. (2002) Prevalence and correlates of alcohol-induced blackouts among college students: Results of an e-mail survey. *J. Am. College Health;* 51,117-131.

White AM, Signer ML, Kraus CL, Swartzwelder HS. (2004) Experimental aspects of alcohol-induced blackouts among college students. *The American Journal of Drug and Alcohol Abuse;* Vol.30, No.1, pp. 205-224.

White, W, Kurtz, E. (2006) The varieties of recovery experience. *International Journal of Self Help and Self Care,* 2006; 3: 21–61.

Williamson, A., Darke, S., Ross, J., Teesson, M., (2006). The effect of persistence of cocaine use on 12-month outcomes for the treatment of heroin dependence. *Drug Alcohol Depend.* 81, 293–300.

Windle, M. and Scheit, D. M. (2004) Alcoholic subtypes: are two sufficient? *Addiction.* 99, 1508–1519.

Witkiewitz K, Marlatt GA, Walker DD. (2005) Mindfulnessbased relapse prevention for alcohol use disorders: The meditative tortoise wins the race. *Journal of Cognitive Psychotherapy;* 19: 211–230.

Wurmser L. (1985) Denial and split identity: timely issues in the psychoanalytic psychotherapy of compulsive drug users. *Journal of Substance Abuse Treatment;* 2: 89-96.

Wurmser L. (1987) Flight from conscience: experiences with the psychoanalytic treatment of compulsive drug abusers. *Journal of Substance Abuse Treatment;* 4: 169-179.

Yan YM, Xu H , Li DY. (2000) Questionnaire analysis on physical-mental health state in 169 cases heroin addicts. *Guizhou Medical Journal;* 24 (5): 318.

Yan YQ, Liu YY, Zeng YF, Cui YW, Lei JW, Wang ZZ. (2008) Evaluation of Effectiveness of Integrated Intervention Program in Improving Drug Addicts' Psychological Health. *Biomedical and Environmental Sciences;* 21: 75-84.

Young, R. M., & Knight, R. G. (1989). The Drinking Expectancy Questionnaire: A revised measure of alcohol-related beliefs. *Journal of Psychopathology and Behavioral Assessment.* 11, 99–112.

Young, R. McD., Oei, T.P.S. & Crook, C.M. (1991). Development of a Drinking Self Efficacy Scale. *Journal of Psychopathology and Behavioral Assessment,* 13(1), 1-15.

Yücel M; Lubman D; Solowij N; Brewer W. (2009) Understanding drug addiction: a neuropsychological perspective. *Australian and New Zealand Journal of Psychiatry,* 41:12,957 — 968.

Zador S, Sunjic D. (2000) Deaths in methadone maintenance treatment in New South Wales, Australia, 1990–1995. *Addiction.* 95:77–86.

Zinn S, Stein R, Swartzwelder S. (2004) Executive functioning early in abstinence from alcohol. *Alcoholism: Clinical and Experimental Research;* Vol.28; No 9, pp 1338-1346.

Index

B

C

D

E

F

G

N

O

P

Q

R

S

W

Y